Practical Traditional
Chinese Medicine &
Pharmacology

Basic Theories
and Principles

By Geng Junying and Su Zhihong

 New World Press, Beijing

First Edition 1990
Second Printing 1996

ISBN 7 - 80005 - 114 - 5

Published by:
New World Press
24 Baiwanzhuang Road, Beijing, 100037, China

Distributed by:
China International Book Trading Corporation
35 Chegongzhuang Xilu, Beijing, 100044, China
P.O. Box 399, Beijing, China

Printed in the People's Republic of China

Contents

Preface 1

Introduction 4

Chapter 1
The *Yin-Yang* and Five
Elements Theories 6

Section 1
The Theory of *Yin-Yang* 7

1. The Basic Content of *Yin-Yang* Theory 7
2. The Application of *Yin-Yang* Theory
   to the Field of Traditional Chinese Medicine 11

Section 2
The Five Elements Theory 15

1. The Basic Content of the Five Elements Theory 15
2. Application of the Five Elements Theory
   to Traditional Chinese Medicine 19

Chapter 2
The *Zang-Fu* Theory 24

Section 1
The Five *Zang* Organs 25

1. Heart 25
1,a. Pericardium 27
2. Lung 27
3. Spleen 31
4. Liver 33
5. Kidneys 36

I

5,a. Uterus   40

Section 2
The Six *Fu* Organs   40

1. Gall Bladder   40
2. Stomach   40
3. Small Intestine   41
4. Large Intestine   42
5. Urinary Bladder   42
6. *Sanjiao*   42

Chapte 3
Qi, Blood, and Body Fluid   44

Section 1
Qi   44

1. Primary *Qi* (yuan *qi*)   45
2. Aggregative *qi* (zong *qi*)   45
3. Nutrient *Qi* (ying *qi*)   45
4. Defensive *Qi* (wei *qi*)   45

Section 2
Blood   46

Section 3
Body Fluid   46

Chapter 4
The Theory of Channels
And Collaterals   48

Section 1
The Formation and Functions
of Channels and Collaterals   48

1. Channnels and Collaterals Systems   48

2. Channels and Collaterals Functions   49

Section 2
The Twelve Regular Channels   51

1. The Lung Channel of the Hand Taiyin   51
2. The Large Intestine Channel of the Hang-Yangming   51
3. The Stomach Channel of the Foot-Yangming   52
4. The Spleen Channel of the Foot-Taiyin   57
5. The Heart Channel of the Hand-Shaoyin   58
6. The Small Intestine Channel of the Hand-Taiyang   58
7. The Urinary Bladder Channel of the Foot-Taiyang   59
8. The Kidney Channel of the Foot-Shaoyin   60
9. The Pericardium Channel of the Hand-Jueyin   65
10. The *Sanjiao* Channel of the Hand-Shaoyang   66
11. The Gall Bladder Channel of the Foot-Shaoyang   66
12. The Liver Channel of the Foot-Jueyin   68

Section 3
Pathways, Conjunctures, Exterior-
Interior Relationships and the Order
of *Qi* Flow in the Channels   73

1. Pathways and Conjunctures   73
2. Exterior-Interior Relationships and the Order
   of the *Qi* Flow in the Channels   73

Section 4
Eight Extra Channels   75

1. The Ren Channel   75
2. The Du Channel 80
3. The Chong Channel   80
4. The Dai Channel   81
5. The Yinwei Channel   81
6. The Yangwei Channel   81
7. The Yinqiao Channel   82
8. The Yangqiao Channel   82

Section 5
The Fifteen Collaterals   87

Section 6
The Twelve Divergent Channels   87

Section 7
The Twelve Musculotendinous Regions
of the Regular Channels   89

Section 8
The Twelve Cutaneous Regions
of the Regular Channels   90

Chapter 5
Etiology 91

Section 1
Six Exogenous Factors   92

1. Wind   93
2. Cold   94
3. Summer-Heat   96
4. Damp   97
5. Dryness   99
6. Fire Heat or Mild Heat   99

Section 2
Pestilential Factors   101

Section 3
Seven Emotional Factors   101

Section 4
Other Pathogenic Factors   102

1. Irregular Diet   104

2. Traumatic Injuries and Parasites   104
3. Phlegm-Humor and Blood Stagnation   104

Chapter 6
Methods of Diagnosis   106

Section 1
Inspection   107

1. Observation of the Mind   107
2. Observation of the Complexion   107
3. Observation of the Tongue   109

Section 2
Auscultation and Olfaction   112

1. Listening   112
2. Smelling   113
3. Inquiring   113
4. Palpation   120

Chapter 7
Differentiation of Syndromes   125

Section 1
Differentiation of Syndromes
According to the Eight Principles   126

1. Exterior and Interior   127
2. Cold and Heat   127
3. *Xu* (deficiency) and *Shi* (Excess)   128
4. *Yin* and *Yang*   129

Section 2
Differentiating Syndromes According
to the *Zang-Fu* Organs   131

1. Differentiating Syndromes of the Heart   131

2. Differentiating Syndromes of the Liver **133**
3. Differentiating Syndromes of the Spleen **136**
4. Differentiating Lun Syndromes **138**
5. Differentiating Syndromes of the Kidney **140**
6. Differentiating Syndromes of the Small Intestine **143**
7. Differentiating Syndromes of the Large Intestine **143**
8. Differentiating Syndromes of the Urinary Bladder **144**
9. Differentiating Syndromes of the Stomach **144**
10. Differentiating Gall Bladder Syndromes **145**

Section 3
Differentiating Syndromes According
to the Theories of the Six Channels, Four Stages of
Wei, Qi, Ying and *Xue*, and *Sanjiao* **146**

1. Differentiating Syndromes According
   to Six Channels Theory **147**
2. Differentiating Syndromes According to the Theory
   of *Wei, Qi, Ying,* and *Xue* **153**
3. *Differentiating Syndromes According to the Sanjiao* Theory **158**

Chapter 8
Therapeutic Principles 162

1. The Principle of *Biao* and *Ben* **162**
2. Strengthening the *Zheng Qi* and Dispelling *Xie Qi* **163**
3. Principle of Treatment Based on Climatic and Seasonal Conditions,
   Geographic Localities, and Patient's Personal Conditions **163**
Endnotes 166

Preface

    This series of "Practical Traditional Chinese Medicine and Pharmacology" consists of five separate books: *Basic Theories and Principles*; *Acupuncture and Moxibustion*; *Medicinal Herbs*; *Herbal Formulas*; and *Clinical Experiences*. These books represent a comprehensive and systematic treatment of the theories and practices of traditional Chinese medicine and pharmacology. This series incorporates a practical approach to the study of Chinese medicine through its use of simple explanations and thorough outlines.

    In the first volume, *Basic Theories and Principles*, the Yin-Yang and Five Elements theories are addressed as the basic philosophical elements of traditional Chinese medicine. The theories of physiology, pathology, etiology, diagnostic methodology, and syndrome differentiation in traditional Chinese medicine are explained in a discussion of the *zang-fu* organs (the internal organs) and channels-collaterals. These theories stress the importance of the appropriate holistic treatment according to an accurate diagnosis of the particular complaint. Thus the reader can learn the methods of understanding disease using the vantage point of traditional Chinese medicine and also com-

1

mand a knowledge of its basic theories.

The second volume, *Acupuncture and Moxibustion*, introduces techniques of acupuncture and moxibustion, commonly used acupuncture points, basic laws and methods of selecting points, and details of acupuncture treatment of the common diseases as described in an appendix of typical cases. It enables the reader to learn not only acupuncture techniques for more than forty kinds of diseases and symptoms, but also methods of selecting appropriate points for different symptoms. The third and fourth volumes, *Medicinal Herbs* and *Herbal Formulas*, provide exhaustive and practicable information on individual traditional Chinese medicinal herbs, and formulas of medicinal herbs. The former presents the theory of the Four Properties and Five Flavors of herbal drugs, the theory of ascending and descending, floating and sinking, and direction of action of medicinal herbs. Also discussed is a description of the origin, property, flavor, and classification of three hundred herbs according to their therapeutic action on diseases of specific channels, general therapeutic action, indications, dispensation of herbal prescription, and contraindications. Readers will learn in the fourth volume the original source and ingredients of one hundred fifty commonly used herbal formulas, and their therapeutic actions, indications, and contraindications. By bringing theories, methods, prescriptions, and individual herbs together, they reflect the philosophy of traditional Chinese medicine which applies treatment on the basis of syndrome differentiation. Readers will not only become acquainted with one hundred fifty commonly used herbal formulas, but also with the laws and methods of differentiating syndromes, the principles of constructing herbal prescriptions, and other aspects of traditional Chinese herbal medicine. The fifth volume, *Clinical Experiences*, introduces therapeutic methods of treating common internal disease, gynecology, and pediatrics. It associates practical application of theories, methods, herbal formulas, and individual herbs with clinical methods.

Preface

Moreover, readers can use the fifth volume to learn the basic methods of applying treatment according to syndrome differentiation using the theories of traditional Chinese medicine and pharmacology. This series on traditional Chinese medicine has been compiled by professionals with many years of experience in teaching, scientific research, and clinical treatment. Each volume has been checked and approved by leading authorities in the field of traditional Chinese medicine and pharmacology. These books present the reader with an easy access to state of the art knowledge on Chinese traditional medicine and pharmacology. The information presented in this series is the product of years of combined research and provides a reference for beginners as well as professionals in the field of traditional medicine. At present it is rare to read English editions which completely and systematically introduce traditional Chinese medical philosophies and methodologies with such conciseness. We hope that this series is able to involve interested readers from all over the world in the development and dissemination of this ancient art for the benefit of the human race.

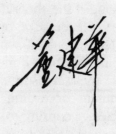

Professor **Dong Jianhua**

Director of the All-China Association
of Traditional Chinese Medicine
Advisor to the Public Health Ministry
of the People's Republic of China

Introduction

The basic theories of traditional Chinese medicine describe the physiology and pathology of the human body, disease etiology, diagnosis, and differentiation of symptom-complexes. This includes the theories of Yin-Yang, Five Elements, *zang-fu*, channels-collaterals, *qi*, blood, body fluid, methods of diagnosis, and differentiation of symptom-complexes.

Traditional Chinese medical theories possess two outstanding features, their holistic point of view, and their application of treatment according to the differentiation of symptom-complexes. According to these traditional viewpoints, the *zang-fu* organs are the core of the human body as an organic entity in which tissues and sense organs are connected through a network of channels and collaterals. This concept is applied extensively to physiology, pathology, diagnosis, and treatment.

The functional physiological activities of the *zang-fu* organs are dissimilar, but they work in coordination. There exists an organic connection between the organs and their related tissues.

Introduction

Pathologically, a dysfunction of the *zang-fu* organs may be reflected on the body surface through the channels and their collaterals. At the same time, diseases of body surface tissues may also affect their related *zang* or *fu* organs. Affected *zang* or *fu* organs may also influence each other through internal connections. Traditional Chinese medical treatment consists of regulating the functions of the *zang-fu* organs in order to correct pathological changes. With acupuncture, treatment is accomplished by stimulating certain areas of the external body.

Not only is the human body an organic whole, but it is also a unified entity within nature, so changes in the natural environment may directly or indirectly affect it. For example, changes of the four seasons, and the alternations of day and night may change the functional condition of the human body, while various geographical environments can influence differences in body constitution, and so on. These factors must be considered when diagnosis and treatment are given. The principles of treatment are expected to accord with the different seasons and environments.

Application of treatment according to the differentiation of syndromes is another characteristic of traditional Chinese medicine. "Differentiation of syndromes" means to analyze the disease condition in order to know its essentials, to identify the causative factors, the location and nature, and to obtain conclusions about the confrontation between pathogenic and antipathogenic factors. In traditional Chinese medicine, differentiation is performed to outline the specific principles and methods of treatment because similar diseases may have different clinical manifestations, while different diseases may share the same syndromes. Treatment in traditional Chinese medicine stresses the differences of syndromes, but not the differences of diseases. Therefore different treatments for the same disease exist and different diseases can be treated by the same method.

Chapter 1
The Yin-Yang and Five Elements Theories

The theories of Yin-Yang and Five Elements were the creation and development of the ancient Chinese through their long and faithful tradition of observing nature's cycles and changes. They held that wood, fire, earth, metal, and water were the basic substances constituting the material world. these five basic substances were considered an indispensable part of daily life. They also noted that the material world is in a constant state of flux due to the dynamic movement and mutual antagonism of *yin* and *yang* factors.

The ancient Chinese applied these two theories in the medical field to explain the physiological activities and pathological changes of the human body, and to serve as a guide to the clinical treatment on the basis of syndrome differentiation. These theories have become an important component of traditional Chinese medicine.

Section 1
The Theory of Yin-Yang

The Yin-Yang theory holds that all phenomena consist of two opposite aspects, *yin* and *yang*, which are variously defined as: up and down, left and right, light and dark, hot and cold, stillness and movement, substance and function, etc. The movements and changes of *yin* and *yang* give impetus to the development of everything or in the words of the *Suwen*, "*Yin* and *yang* are the law of Heaven and Earth, the outline of everything, the parents of change, the origin of birth and destruction...."[1]

Yin and *yang* represent two opposite aspects of every object and its implicit conflict and interdependence. Generally, anything that is moving, ascending, bright, progressing, hyperactive, including functional diseases of the body, pertains to *yang*. The characteristics of stillness, descending, darkness, degeneration, hypoactivity, including organic diseases, pertain to *yin*.

The nature of *yin* and *yang* is relative. According to Yin-Yang theory, everything in the universe can be divided into the two opposite but complementary aspects of *yin* and *yang* and either aspect can again be divided into the two aspects of *yin* and *yang* and so on ad infinitum. For example, day is *yang* and night is *yin*, but morning is understood as being *yang* within *yang*, afternoon is *yin* within *yang*, evening before midnight is *yin* within *yin* and the time after midnight is *yang* within *yin*. As the *Suwen* states, "*Yin* and *yang* could amount to ten in number, be extended to one hundred, to one thousand, to ten thousand and even to the infinite."[2]

1. The Basic Content of Yin-Yang Theory

The Opposition of Yin and Yang

The theory of Yin-Yang holds that every object in the universe consists of two opposite aspects which are in continual mutual restriction and interaction. The alternation of the four seasons is an example. The spring is warm and the summer hot. This is due to the rising of *yang qi* which restricts the autumn cool and the winter cold. Alternately, the coolness of autumn and cold of winter arise because of the ascendancy of *yin* that restricts the spring warmth and summer heat. According to Yin-Yang theory, the seasonal cycle is the outcome of the mutually restrictive and mutually consuming-increasing activities of *yin* and *yang*. Either side of the two opposites always restricts and acts on the other. This process of mutual restriction and interaction is the operation of *yin* and *yang*, without which change would not occur. Thus the two opposites of *yin* and *yang* do not exist as an entity in a still and unconcerned state. They constantly interact with each other, hence the alteration and development of an object.

Yin and Yang Interdependence

Yin and *yang* are at once in opposition and in interdependence. They rely on each other for existence, coexisting in a single entity. Each of the two aspects is the condition for the other's existence and neither can exist in isolation. for example, daytime is *yang*, night is *yin*, without day there would be no night; upper is *yang*, lower is *yin*; left is *yang*, right is *yin*, etc., each pair exists in a state of mutual dependence, and without its opposite it could not exist. The interdependent relationship of *yin* and *yang* is described in the *Suwen*, "*Yin* is installed in the interior as the material foundation for *yang*, while *yang* remains on the exterior as the manifestation of the *yin* function."[3] This is a traditional explanation of the interdependence of *yin* and *yang*.

The Mutual Consuming-Increasing Relationship of Yin and Yang

The *yin* and *yang* aspects within an object are not quiescent, but in a state of constant motion. They can be described as being in a state where the lessening of *yin* leads to an increase of *yang*, or vise versa. Taking the transformation of the seasons as an example, in terms of the Yin-Yang theory, the process of transition from winter cold through spring warmth into summer heat demonstrates the process of a lessening of *yin* leading into an increasing of *yang*. While the transition from the heat of summer to the cold of winter is the lessening of *yang* leading to an increasing of *yin*.

Regarding the human body's functional activities, which are considered *yang*, the consumption of nutrient substances, which are considered *yin*, results in the lessening of *yin* to the increase of *yang*. As the metabolism of nutrient substances (*yin*) exhausts the functional energy (*yang*) to a certain extent, this is understood as a lessening of *yang* to the increase of *yin*. Under normal conditions the mutual consuming and increasing of *yin* and *yang* maintain a relative balance. Under abnormal conditions there is an excess or insufficiency of either *yin* or *yang* which leads to the occurrence of disease.

Yin and Yang's Mutual Transforming Relationship

In certain circumstances and at a certain stage of development, each of the two aspects of *yin* and *yang*, within an object, will transform from *yin* into *yang* and from *yang* into *yin*. The mutual consuming-increasing of *yin* and *yang* is a process of quantitative change, and the mutual transformation of *yin* and *yang* is a process of qualitative change. The *Suwen* comments, "Extreme cold will bring about heat, and extreme heat will induce cold..." furthermore, "Excessive *yin* may cause *yang* syndromes or tend to be transformed into *yang* and vice versa."[4] These are the features and conditions of the mutual transformation of *yin* and *yang*.

The mutual transformation of *yin* and *yang* is often seen during the development of a disease. For example, if a patient has a constant high fever, which is suddenly lowered, accompanied by a pale complexion, cold limbs, extremely feeble pulse (the danger symptoms of *yin* cold syndromes), we may say that the disease has transformed from a *yang* syndrome into a *yin*

The Yin-Yang and Five Elements Theories

○ *Yang*

● *Yin*

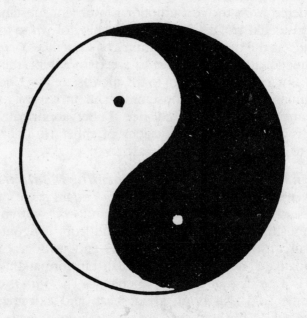

Fig. 1. The Traditional Figure of the *yin* and *yang*

syndrome. Under these circumstances, proper emergency treatment should warm the limbs to make the pulse normal. The *yang qi* will recover, and the danger will be removed. Thus *yin* syndromes can change into *yang* syndromes. Clinical practice provides other examples of the mutual transformation of *yin and yang*. It is common in clinical practice to have exterior syndromes transform into interior syndromes or vice versa and *shi* (excess) syndromes may change into *xu* (deficiency) syndromes or vice versa.

The above-mentioned relationships of mutual opposing, depending, consuming-increasing, and transforming of *yin* and *yang* are the basic content of Yin-Yang theory. Furthermore, these four relationships between *yin* and *yang* are not so isolated from each other but interconnect with and interact upon each other. (See *Fig.* 1)

2. The Application of Yin-Yang Theory to the Field of Traditional Chinese Medicine

The theory of *yin* and *yang* is used extensively in traditional Chinese medicine to explain the histological structure, physiological function, and pathological changes of the human body, and to serve as a guide for diagnosis and treatment.

The Anatomical and Histological Structure of the Human Body

The Yin-Yang theory asserts that the human body is an organic whole, and there exists an organic connection between all tissues and structures. Yet, at the same time, each of them can be divided into the opposite aspects of *yin* and *yang*.

Viewing the body as a whole, the portion above the waist pertains to *yang* and that below belongs to *yin*; the exterior of the body is associated with *yang*, while the interior is associated with *yin*; the back is considered *yang* and the front, *yin*; the lateral aspect is *yang* and the medial, *yin*.

11

The *zang-fu* organs also have *yin* and *yang* aspects, the six *fu* organs are considered *yang* while the *zang* organs are *yin*. Each of the *zang-fu* organs itself can again be divided into *yin* or *yang*; for example, heart *yin* and heart *yang* or kidney *yin* and kidney *yang*. However complex, all human body structures and tissues can be generalized and explained by the *yin-yang* relationship. As the *Suwen* says, "Man has physical shape which is inseparable from *yin* and *yang*."

The Physiological Functions of the Human Body
The Yin-Yang theory considers the normal vital activities of the human body to be the result of the relative balance between *yin* and *yang*. In traditional Chinese medicine, the physiological functions of the organs and their substances are inseparably related to *yin* and *yang*. For example, the activities (*yang*) of a particular organ are based on that organ's substance (*yin*), and when either of these aspects is absent, the other cannot function. Thus the result of physiological activities is to constantly promote the transformation of *yang* into *yin* essence. If *yin* and *yang* cannot maintain relative balance and interaction, they will separate from each other ending the life that depends upon them. As the *Suwen* says, "When *yin* keeps balance with *yang* and both maintain a normal condition of *qi*, then health will be high-spirited. A separation of *yin* and *yang* will lead to the exhaustion of essential *qi*."

The Pathological Changes of the Human Body
The Yin-Yang theory holds that disease is a result of an imbalance between *yin* and *yang* which leads to the hyperactivity or hypoactivity of *yin* and *yang*. The occurrence and the development of a disease are also related to *zheng qi* (body resistance or antipathogenic factors) and *xie qi* (pathogenic factors). The Yin-Yang theory can be used to generalize the interacting relations between body resistance and antipathogenic factors. Pathogenic factors are divided into *yang*-natured pathogenic factors and *yin*-natured pathogenic factors, while

zheng qi includes *yin* essence and *yang qi*. *Yang* pathogenic factors may bring about hypoactivity of bodily *yang* which leads to injury of *yin*; a heat syndrome results. If the disease is caused by *yin* pathogenic factors, it may give rise to hypoactivity of *yin* followed by the injury of *yang*; a cold syndrome will result. When *yang* is deficient it fails to restrict *yin* in the balanced relationship between the two giving rise to *xu* (deficiency) which is a cold syndrome. The *xu* heat symptom complex, however, is caused by a *yin* deficiency and *yang* excess. Pathological changes of diseases are varied, but can be generally explained in terms of *yin-yang* imbalance: *yin* excess causes cold syndromes, *yang* preponderance leads to heat syndromes, *yang* deficiency causes cold syndromes, and *yin* deficiency leads to heat syndromes.

Diagnosis of Diseases

The basic causative factor of disease is an imbalance between *yin* and *yang*. Therefore, no matter how intricate and volatile the clinical manifestations are, they can still be summarized into two categories: *yin* syndromes and *yang* syndromes. A correct diagnosis depends upon a clear classification of *yin* and *yang* syndromes or in the words of the *Suwen*, "If one is good at diagnosis, they should differentiate the *yin* from *yang* after the observation of color (of complexion, tongue, urine, stool, etc.) and feeling the pulse."[7] The four diagnostic methods (inspection, auscultation and olfaction, inquiry, and palpation) also use *yin* and *yang*, for example: interior, *xu* (deficiency), and cold syndromes are considered *yin*; exterior, *shi* (excess), and heat syndromes are considered *yang*; bright color is *yang*, dim color is *yin*; a sonorous voice indicates *yang*, a low voice is *yin*; feeble and weak respiration is *yin*, coarse breathing is *yang*; superficial, rapid, and forceful pulses are *yang*, slow, deep feeble, and weak pulses are *yin*.

Applications in Clinical Treatment

Since imbalance and fluctuation of *yin* and *yang* are considered the basic causative factors of disease occurrence and development, treatment must readjust *yin* and *yang* to their basic state of relative balance. For example, if pathogenic heat, a *yang* disease causative factor, is overabundant, it consumes the *yin* fluid and affects the superabundant *yang* of the body. In this case, the cold method for heat syndromes (for example, the use of herbs with a "cold" nature to cure "heat" illnesses) is the prescribed treatment. If pathogenic cold is in excess, it will damage the *yang qi* and exert influence on the body's remaining *yin*. In this case, the heat method for cold syndromes (for example, the use of herbs with a "hot" nature to cure "cold" illnesses) is used. Conversely, in cases where *yang* excess is caused by insufficient *yin* fluid failing to restrict *yang* or where *yin* preponderance is due to *yang qi* deficiency being unable to control *yin*, then treatment should reinforce the insufficient *yin* or *yang*. The general principle is, "Treat *yin* for *yang* diseases, and treat *yang* for *yin* disorders."

In medical treatment, the theory of *yin* and *yang* is not only used to decide the principles of treatment. This theory is also generally applied to the properties, flavor, and action of Chinese herbal medicine as a guide to the clinical administration of herbs. For example, drugs with cold, cool, or moist properties are classified as *yin* and drugs with the opposite properties are classified as *yang*. Herbs with sour, bitter, or salty flavors are *yin*, while those with pungent, sweet, or insipid flavors are *yang*. Drugs with an astringent or descending action are *yin* and those with an ascending and dispersing action are *yang*. In clinical treatment, we should determine the principles of treatment based on an analysis of the *yin* and *yang* conditions present in terms of their different *yin-yang* properties and actions. The goal of clinical treatment is to restore a healthy *yin-yang* properties and actions. The goal of clinical treatment is to restore a healthy *yin-yang* balance in the patient.

Section 2
The Five Elements Theory

The Five Elements theory posits wood, fire, earth, metal, and water as the basic elements of the material world. These elements are in constant movement and change. Moreover, the complex connections between material objects are explained through the relationship of interdependence and mutual restraint that governs the five elements. In traditional Chinese medicine Five Elements theory is used to interpret the relationship between the physiology and pathology of the human body and the natural environment.

1. The Basic Content of the Five Elements Theory

The Categorization of Things
The ancient physicians used the Five Elements theory to study extensively the connections between the physiology and pathology of the *zang-fu* organs and tissues and the natural environment. By adopting the methodology of "comparing similarity to expose phenomenon," the ancient Chinese attributed different phenomena to the categories of the five elements. On the basis of the phenomena's different characteristics, functions, and forms, the complex links between physiology and pathology as well as the correlation between the human body and the natural environment were explained.

Five Elements theory assigns each of the five elements a series of abstract generalizations and then applies them to the classification of all phenomena. Wood, for example, involves the aspects of germination, extension, softness, and harmony. It is then inferred that anything with those characteristics should be included in the category of the wood element. As for the rest of the five elements: fire involves the aspects of heat and flaring; earth involves the aspects of growing, nourishing, and changing;

metal is associated with cleaning up, killing, strength, and firmness; and water is associated with cold, moisture, and downward flowing. As in the case of wood, the aspects of the other five elements are used to categorize all material objects in terms of one of the particular five elements. *Table* 1 shows the five categories of objects and phenomena according to five elements classification.

Table 1.

Categorization of Objects and Phenomena According to the Five Elements

Objects & Phenomena	Elements				
	Wood	Fire	Earth	Metal	Water
Nature					
Tones	Jiao	Zheng	Gong	Shang	Yu
Flavors	Sour	Bitter	Sweet	Pungent	Salty
Color	green	Red	Yellow	White	Black
Changes	Germinate	Grow	Transform	Reap	Store
Climate	Wind	Summer Humid	Dampness	Dryness	Coldness
Directions	East	South	Center	West	North
Seasons	Spring	Summer	Late Summer	Autumn	Winter
Human Body					
Zang Fu	Liver	Heart	Spleen	Lung	Kidney
	Gall Bladder	S. Intestine	Stomach	L. Intestine	Urinary
Senses	Eye	Tongue	Mouth	Nose	Ear
Tissue	Tendon	Vessel	Muscle	Skin& Hair	Bone
Emotions	Anger	Joy	Thinking	Melancholy	Fear
Sound	Shout	Laugh	Sing	Cry	Mourn

The Mutual Generation, Mutual Subjugation, Extreme Subjugation, and Counter Subjugation Relationships of the Five Elements

The Five Elements theory asserts that between each of the elements there exists the close relationships of mutual generation, mutual subjugation, extreme subjugation, and counter subjugation. The theory explains the interrelatedness of all things through the use of those close relationships.

Mutual generation means multiplication and promotion, while mutual subjugation means mutual restriction and restraint. The order of mutual generation among the five elements is that wood generates fire, fire generates earth, earth generates metal, metal generates water, and water generates wood. In this way generation is circular and endless. In the mutual generating relation of the five elements, each of the elements has the property of "being generated" and "generating." The one which generates is the "mother," the one which is generated is the "son." This is know as the "mother-son relationship." Each of the five elements has this type of mutual generating relationship with the other.

According to the order of mutual subjugation, however, wood subjugates earth, metal subjugates wood, etc. Each of the five elements also shares this subjugational relationship with the other. This relationship has the properties of "being subjugated" and of "subjugating." The former means that my ability is inferior to the object, while the later denotes my superiority to the object. Therefore, the mutual subjugating relationship among the five elements is also known as the relationship of "being superior to" and "being inferior to" another element.

Mutual generation and mutual subjugation are two aspects which cannot be separated. If there is no generation, then there is no birth and growth. If there is no subjugation, then there is no change and development for maintaining normal harmonious relations. As the *Leijing tuyi* says, "If there is no generation, then there is no growth and development. If there is no restric-

17

tion, then endless growth and development will become harmful."[8] Thus the movement and change of all things exists through their mutual generating and subjugating relationships. These relationships are the basis of the never ending circulation of natural elements.

Extreme subjugation and counter subjugation are the pathological conditions of the normal mutual generation and subjugation relationships. Extreme subjugation denotes that the subjugation of one of the five elements to another surpasses the normal level. For example, if there is hyperactivity of the wood element, it will subjugate the earth element. The latter elements is made weak and insufficient.

Counter subjugation means that one of the five elements subjugates the other opposite to the normal mutual subjugation order. For example, when metal is weak and insufficient, it leads to the hyperactivity of wood. The latter will then counter subjugate the former. In the *Suwen* it says:

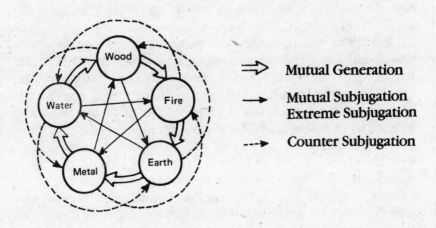

Fig. 2. The Inter-Relationship of the Five Elements

When the *qi* of one of the five elements is excessive, it will subjugate its subjugated element (such as wood subjugating earth) and counter subjugate the subjugating element (such as wood counter subjugating metal).[9]

Moreover, the Five Elements theory recognizes a correlation between those things which are related to a particular element. As the *Suwen* points out, "The East generates wind, wind generates wood, wood generates sour, sour generates liver, liver generates tendons...."[10] According to Five Elements theory, each element has its own repertory of relationships among the objects that compose the physical world. The theory of Five Elements is therefore the theoretical basis of the unique bond between man and nature. (See *Fig. 2*)

2. Application of the Five Elements Theory to Traditional Chinese Medicine

The Five Elements theory is applied to the physiology and pathology of the human body by using the relationships of generation and subjugation to guide clinical diagnosis and treatment.

The Physiological Functions and Interrelationships of the Five Zang Organs

Physiologically the Five Elements theory explains the unity of the mutual relationships between the *zang-fu* organs and body tissues as well as between the human body and nature. The physiological activities of the five *zang* organs can be classified according to the different characteristics of the five elements. For example, the liver is said to preside over the vigorous flow of *qi* and also has the function of ensuring free *qi* circulation. Since these characteristics are similar to the properties of wood, the liver is categorized as wood in the scheme of the five elements.

Heart *yang* has a warming action so it belongs to the category of the fire element. The spleen is the source of transformation of essential substances and is associated with the earth element's characteristics of growth and transformation. The lung has clearing and descending properties and is associated with the metal element's characteristics of clearing and astringency. The kidney has the function of controlling water metabolism and storing essence and is associated with the water element's characteristics of moistening and flowing downward.

The Five Elements theory is also used to describe the correlations of physiological functions between *zang-fu* organs and body tissues. There are both generating and subjugating relationships among the five *zang* organs. The generating relationships are: the essence of kidney (represented by the water element) nourishes the liver; the liver (represented by the wood element) stores the blood in order to support the heart; the heat of the heart (represented by the fire element) warms the spleen; the spleen (represented by the earth element) transforms and transports the essential nutrients to replenish the lung; and the clearing and descending functions of the lung (represented by the metal element) assist the flowing of kidney water.

The subjugating relationships among the same organs are as follows: the clearing and descending functions of the lung (metal element) can restrict the hyperactivity of liver *yang*; the unobstructed flowing of liver (wood element) *qi* is capable of removing the stagnation of the spleen (earth element); the transportation and transformation of spleen is able to subdue the overflowing of kidney water; and the nourishing and moistening function of kidney (water element) can prevent the strong flaring up of heart fire. The *yang* heat of the heart (fire element) can control the hyperactivity of the lung's clearing and descending functions.

Furthermore, the Five Elements theory is employed to express the mutual relationships between the human body with the seasons, climates, and flavors. For example, while the wood element is associated with East, spring, wind, sour, etc., it is also connected with the liver, tendons, and eyes of the human body. In this way the Five Elements theory gives expression to a holistic view of the relationship between the human body and its natural environment.

Five Elements Theory and Pathological Influences on the Zang-Fu Organs

Five Elements theory is not only used to correlate the functions of the *zang-fu* organs, but also to demonstrate their mutual pathological influence. To denote the mutual influence of the *zang-fu* organs in pathological changes the concepts of extreme subjugation and counter subjugation are used. For example, liver disease may affect the spleen because wood over-subjugates earth, while spleen illness may affect the liver as earth counter subjugates wood. Diseases of the liver and spleen interact with each other. Liver disease may also influence the heart, this is a "mother affecting son" illness. If the liver disease is transmitted to the lung, this is categorized as wood counter subjugating metal. If it is transmitted to the kidney, then it is considered a "son affecting mother" illness. the other *zang* organs follow suit. Thus the application of the Five Elements theory in explaining the complicated interaction between the *zang* organs can be summed up by these four relationships: extreme subjugation, counter subjugation, mother affecting son illness, and son affecting mother illness.

Use of the Five Elements Theory in the Diagnosis and Treatment of Disease

Abnormal changes of the internal organ's functions and interrelationships can be detected by external appearances. Thus changes in a patient's complexion, voice, sense of taste, pulse, etc. can be used to diagnose disease. According to the Five Elements theory the five *zang* organs have certain connections with the "five colors," "five tones," and "five tastes" as well as changes in the pulse.[11] Therefore, in the clinical diagnosis of a

21

disease, the data collected by the four diagnostic methods (inspection, auscultation and olfaction, inquiring, and palpation) should be analyzed according to the properties and changing laws of mutual generation and subjugation, extreme subjugation, and counter subjugation of the Five Elements theory. For example, a blue complexion accompanied with a preference for food of a sour taste and a wiry pulse, suggests liver disease. A flushed face accompanied by a bitter taste in the mouth and a forceful pulse suggests heart disease with the symptom-complex of heart-fire flaring up. A patient with insufficient spleen *qi* may have a blue complexion implying wood's (i.e., liver) extreme subjugation of earth (i.e., spleen). If a patient is suffering from heart trouble and has a dark complexion, it may be explained as water (i.e., kidney) subjugating fire.

The occurrence and development of a disease is sometimes related to the abnormality of the mutual generation and subjugation relationships. Therefore, clinical treatment should not only concentrate on the diseased *zang* organ, but also be concerned with readjusting the relationships between the particular *zang* or *fu* organs in accordance with Five Elements theory. For example, the *Nanjing* says, "When the liver is diseased, the liver will transmit to the spleen, and so one should replenish the *qi* of the spleen."[12] This reflects the clinical application of five element's extreme subjugation theory. The laws of mutual generation and subjugation and extreme subjugation and counter subjugation have been applied by subsequent generations of traditional Chinese medicine practitioners to create more methods of treatment such as "cultivating the earth in order to generate metal," "nourishing the water to conserve wood," "supporting the earth to restrict wood," etc.

The *yin-yang* and Five Elements theories represent the world outlook and methodology of the ancient Chinese for their understanding and explanation of nature. The application of these two theories to Chinese medicine consists of viewing the phenomena and laws of nature and applying them to the study

22

of the physiological activities and pathological changes of the human body and its interrelationships. The theory of Yin-Yang explains the dynamics of physical objects through a consideration of their contrary, mutual depending, consuming-increasing and transforming relationships. Normal human physiological activities are understood as the relative balance and harmonization between *yin* and *yang*. When *yin* and *yang* lose their relative balance and coordination, disease occurs. The theories of Yin-Yang and the Five Elements are used together as a guide to clinical diagnosis and treatment.

Chapter 2
The Zang-Fu Theory

The *zang-fu* theory explains the physiological function, pathological changes, and mutual relationships of every *zang* and *fu* organ. In traditional Chinese medicine the *zang* and *fu* organs are not simply anatomical substances, but more importantly represent the generalization of the physiology and pathology of certain systems of the human body.

Zang and *fu* consist of the five *zang* and six *fu* organs. The five *zang* organs are the heart (including the pericardium), lung, spleen, liver, and kidney. The six *fu* organs are the gall bladder, stomach, large intestine, small intestine, urinary bladder and the *sanjiao* (three areas of the body cavity). *Zang* and *fu* are classified by the different features of their functions. The five *zang* organs mainly manufacture and store essence: *qi*, blood, and body fluid. The six *fu* organs mainly receive and digest food, absorb nutrient substances, transmit and excrete wastes. As the *Suwen* says:

The five *zang* organs store up essential *qi* and regulate its outflow. The six *fu* organs transform and transport substances without storing them and for this reason they may be over-filled but cannot be filled to capacity.[13]

There is another category of organs called the extraordinary *fu* organs which include the brain, marrow, bone, vessels, gall bladder, and uterus. They are named *fu* but their functions are similar to that of the five *zang* organs. Since their physiological functions and pathological changes are closely connected with the *zang-fu* organs they will be discussed below under the specific *zang* or *fu* organ.

Section 1
The Five *Zang* Organs

1.1. Heart

The main physiological functions and indicators of the heart are: 1) domination of blood and vessels, and facial complexion; 2) control of the mind; and 3) opening into the tongue. The heart has an "exterior" (*biao*) and "interior" (*li*) relationship with the small intestine.

Dominating Blood and Vessels, and Facial Complexion
The heart dominates the blood and vessels indicating its function of promoting blood circulation. In the *Suwen*, it says, "... the heart is in charge of the blood vessels...."[14] The vessels are the pathways of blood circulation while the heart is the motive power of blood circulation. Only if there is ample heart *qi* can the blood circulate incessantly in the vessels to nourish the whole body. The heart, blood, and vessels are interrelated. Because of the rich distribution of blood vessels in the facial

region, the color and luster of the complexion usually reflects the sufficiency or insufficiency of the blood supply and heart *qi*. If the heart blood supply is sufficient, then the pulse beats normally and forcefully and the facial complexion is rosy with luster. If the heart *qi* is insufficient, the vessels will be empty, the pulse feeble and weak or irregular and the facial complexion pale. Insufficient heart *qi* may lead to blood stagnation manifested by a blue complexion. So in the *Suwen* it says, "The heart is the root of life, ... its luster is manifested in the face, it fills up the blood vessels...."[15]

Controlling the Mind

Mind here indicates spirit, consciousness, and thinking. Traditional Chinese medicine considers that mind refers to the five *zang* organs, especially the heart. so in the *Lingshu* it says, "The organ that is responsible for the performance of activities is the heart."[16] This means the process of thinking is accomplished by the heart. Blood is the main foundation for mental activities, thus the function of heart controlling the mind is closely related to the function of heart dominating the blood and the vessels. If there is plenty of heart blood, the mind is clear, thinking is nimble, and one is full of vim and vigor. If heart blood is insufficient, it will lead to the pathological changes of heart-mind manifested by palpitation, insomnia, dream disturbed sleep, poor memory, restlessness, etc. If heat in the blood disturbs the heart-mind, there will be delirium, coma, etc.

Opening into the Tongue

One of the branches of the heart channel directly connects with the tongue. So physiologically the tongue has a close relationship with the heart. The *qi* and the heart blood all flow up to the tongue in order to assist its normal physiological functions. If there is a pathological change in the heart, it will be reflected in the changes of the tongue. For example, an insufficient supply of heart blood may be manifested by pale tongue proper; heart fire flaring up is reflected by red tongue proper, or even by ulcers of the tongue; blood stagnation in the vessels in presented by a purple tongue or purpura; pathogenic heat invading the pericardium or pathogenic phlegm obstructing the heart orifice, will produce coma, delirium, and stiffness of the tongue. Thus it is said, "The heart opens to the tongue," or "The tongue is the sprout of the heart."

1.2. Pericardium

The pericardium is called *xinbaoluo* in Chinese. Structurally it is a membrane surrounding the heart, and physiologically it protects the heart. When exogenous pathogenic factors attack the heart, the pericardium is affected first. The *Lingshu* notes, "Therefore the pathogenic factors that intend to attack the heart must first attack the pericardium."[17] Clinically the symptoms of pathogenic invasion of the pericardium are the same as if the heart was ill. If pathogenic heat attacks the heart, the symptoms are unconsciousness, delirium, etc. If pathogenic phlegm causes mental confusion, unconsciousness or mental disorder, it is known as "pathogenic phlegm obstructing the heart orifice."

2. Lung

The lung is situated in the chest, connects with the throat and opens into the nose. Its main physiological functions and indicators are: 1) dominating *qi* and controlling respiration; 2) dominating the dispersion and descent of *qi*; 3) regulating water passages; and 4) connecting externally with skin and hair. It also has an exterior and interior relationship with the large intestine.

Dominating Qi and Controlling Respiration
This function is composed of two aspects, dominating the *qi* (air) of respiration and controlling respiration. It is the organ where the respiratory air is internally and externally exchanged; clean *qi* from the environment is drawn in and exchanged for

waste *qi*. The other aspect of the lung's function has a close relationship with the formation of collective (*zong*) *qi* which is the combination of essential *qi* transformed from water and food with the inhaled *qi* of the lung. Collective *qi* accumulates in the chest, then flows up to the throat to control respiration. Since all the blood vessels lead to the lung, collective *qi* is distributed throughout the body to nourish the tissues and organs in maintaining the body's normal functional activities. If the lung function is normal, there is an unobstructed circulation of *qi*, with even and harmonious breathing. If there is a deficiency of lung *qi*, there will be feeble respiration, uneven breathing, weak speech, lassitude, etc.

Dominating the Function of Dispersion and Descent

The function of dispersion and descent involves the distribution of *qi*, blood, and body fluid to the *zang-fu* organs, the channel-collaterals, muscles, skin, and hair. Descending function means that lung *qi* is clear and descends. The lung is situated in the upper *jiao* (thoracic cavity) and its *qi* normally flows downward. If lung *qi* fails to descend and instead ascends, then the *qi* will pool together in the lung and be manifested by stuffy chest, cough, asthma, etc.

The two functions of dispersion and descent, although opposite to each other, act in unison. If the dispersing function is not normal, the lung *qi* will not flow downward and vice versa. Harmonious, downward flowing of lung *qi* allows for an unobstructed respiratory tract, uniform breathing, and provides a normal exchange of air in the lung. In this way the lung can distribute *qi*, blood, and body fluid to the entire body, transport waste water down to the urinary bladder, transform it into urine and excrete it.

In pathology, the two functions of dispersion and descent affect each other. If external pathogenic factors attack the exterior of the body, then the lung *qi* fails to spread. This leads to pathological changes like cough and asthma due to the failure of descending lung *qi*. If pathogenic phlegm obstructs the lung, it will bring about an abnormal flowing of lung *qi* leading to pathological changes such as cough, fullness of chest, and gurgling with sputum.

Dominating the Skin and Hair and Regulating Water Passages

Here the skin and hair represent the entire body surface including skin, sweat gland pores, and hire which act as a barrier against the invasion of exogenous pathogenic factors. In this way the lung is understood to have a close connection with the skin and hair. Through the dispersing function of the lung the essentials of food and water are transported to the body surface in order to nourish the skin, hair, and muscles. The lung also spreads defensive (*wei*) *qi* to the body's surface, "warms the tissues between the skin and muscles, replenishes the skin, nourishes the muscles, and regulates the opening and closing of the pores." Therefore the lung has the ability to protect the organic body by defending against the invasion of exogenous pathogenic factors.

Pathologically there is an mutual influencing relationship between the lung, and skin and hair. For example, the invasion of exogenous pathogenic factors proceeds from the skin and hair to the lung. The manifestations are aversion to cold, fever, nasal obstruction, nasal discharge, cough, or even asthma. These are signs of the lung's failure to spread defensive *qi* to the body surface. If lung *qi* is weak and deficient, defensive *qi* is not dispersed and the essential nutrients to the skin and hair are not distributed. This not only causes rough skin and dry hair, but also hypoactivity of the defensive *qi*.

The organic body is easily attacked by external pathogenic factors. Defensive *qi* controls the opening and closing of the pores. When there is lung *qi* deficiency the body surface will be weak and manifests the symptom of spontaneous sweating. If external pathogenic cold attacks the body's exterior the lung will lose its function of dispersing and descending and the pores will close not allowing the formation of sweat.

Regulating the water passages means that the lung regulates water circulation and excretion, and keeps the water passages clear. The lung's dispersing function circulates throughout the body the nutrients which have been removed from food and water. Part of the fluid is discharged as sweat and by the descending function of the lung. Another part of the fluid is continually sent down to the kidney and then, by the *qi* function of the kidney, sent to the urinary bladder to be discharged. Thus the lung is also known as the "upper source of water."

Opening into the Nose

The nose is the gateway of respiration. Clear, unobstructed nasal breathing and smelling rely upon the good functioning of lung *qi*. Since the nose is the opening of the lung, it will also be a passage for the invasion of external pathogenic heat which may attack the lung. Pathologically the lung also has a close relation with the nose. For example, if external pathogenic wind and cold block the lung, it will cause a dysfunction of lung dispersion manifested by stuffy nose, nasal discharge, dull olfaction, etc. If pathogenic heat accumulates in the lung there will be nasal discomfort caused by coarse breathing or dyspnea. In treating this condition, the dispersing method with pungent medicinal herbs is used to act on the lung and nose. Acupuncture stimulation is applied on ear acupoint "lung" to treat nasal polypus, chronic rhinitis, etc. The above-mentioned facts demonstrate the close relationship between the lung and the nose. The throat is also a gateway of respiration, and a vocal organ. The lung channel passes through the throat, so smooth *qi* flow and a clear voice are directly affected by the functions of lung *qi*. Hence when there is a pathological change of the lung, it will cause hoarseness of voice, sore throat, or other pathological changes.

3. Spleen

The spleen is located in the middle *jiao* (abdominal cavity). Its main physiological functions and indicators are: 1) governing transportation and transformation; 2) controlling blood; 3) dominating the muscles and four limbs; 4) opening into the mouth, and lip complexion. The spleen has an exterior and interior relationship with the stomach.

Governing Transportation and Transformation

This function includes the transportation and transformation of water, and of essential nutrients.

If the spleen's transportation and transformation functions are sound then the functions of digestion, absorption and transportation will work normally. Otherwise, abdominal distension, diarrhea, lassitude, emaciation, malnutrition, and other symptoms may occur.

The spleen is also involved in water metabolism. When the spleen transports nutrient substances, it simultaneously distributes water to every tissue of the body carrying out its functions of nourishment and moistening. From the spleen, water is also sent down to the kidney and excreted from the urinary bladder. The whole process of distribution and metabolism of water is jointly accomplished by the lung's dispersing and descending functions and the spleen's transportation and transformation functions. If the spleen fails to transport and transform the water it will lead to various pathological changes. If water accumulates inside the body, it will turn into an inflammatory mucus (phlegm-humor); if it is retained in the skin and muscle, it becomes a swelling (edema); if the water retention is in the intestines, it will cause diarrhea; if it is in the abdominal cavity, it will result in serious fluid accumulation (ascites). In the *Suwen* it says, "... various kinds of diseases caused by dampness with swelling and fullness belong to the spleen."[18]

Since the functions of transportation and transformation of

essential nutrients as well as water are interrelated, their pathological manifestations often accompany each other.

Controlling Blood

The spleen regulates blood circulation inside the blood vessels. If there is a *qi* deficiency in the spleen, then its function of controlling the blood is lost and the blood flows outside of the vessels. This is evidenced by various hemorrhagic symptoms and diseases, such as chronic uterine bleeding.

In order to control the blood, the spleen uses *ying* (nutrient) *qi*, a form of blood *qi*, which it produces. *Qi* behaves as the "commander" of the blood and, at the same time, conserves the blood. Therefore the hemorrhagic symptoms and diseases caused by the failure of spleen controlling blood are actually the results of *qi* failing to conserve blood.

Dominating the Muscles and Four Limbs

The spleen transports and transforms nutrient substances to nourish the muscles. If this function is normal, there will be sufficient nutrition. Any abnormality of transportation and transformation will certainly affect muscle tissue quality. The *Suwen* records, "The spleen is in charge of the muscles."[19]

The normal movements and functions of the four limbs are also closely related to spleen *qi*. When there is sufficient spleen *qi*, the *yang qi* distributes ample nutrient substances all over the body so that the muscles are well nourished and the four limbs are strong and able to move freely. Otherwise if the spleen fails to transport and transform the *yang qi* and nutrient substances, there will be malnutrition of the muscles characterized by muscular atrophy, weakness of the four limbs, etc. Therefore, building up the spleen is the usual clinical treatment for *wei* syndromes of the four limbs.

Opening into the Mouth and Lip Complexion

The appetite and sense of taste are closely related to the transportation and transformation functions of the spleen. If these functions are healthy, then there will be good appetite and a normal sense of taste. If those functions are abnormal, there will be a lack of appetite. A greasy and sweet taste in the mouth is caused by damp obstruction in the spleen. In the *Suwen* it says, "Spleen *qi* is in communication with the mouth, and when the spleen functions harmoniously, the mouth will be able to taste the flavors of the five cereals."[20]

Since the spleen dominates the muscles and opens into the mouth, the strength or weakness of the transporting and transforming functions are reflected in the lips. If the spleen *qi* is not healthy, those functions will be abnormal, a condition which is characterized by yellowish and lusterless lips.

4. Liver

The liver's main physiological functions and indicators are: 1) storing blood; 2) creating unrestrained conditions for *qi*; 3) controlling the tendons and the luster reflected in the nails; and 4) opening into the eye.

Storing Blood

The liver stores blood and regulates the volume of blood circulation according to the needs of various tissues and organs. during rest the amount of blood required by the body decreases and the surplus is stored in the liver. During vigorous activity blood is released from the liver to increase the volume of circulating blood. As *Wang Bin's Annotations on the Suwen* notes, "The liver stores blood, the heart circulates blood. When the body moves blood circulates in the channels, when at rest it flows back to the liver."[21] If the liver's blood storage function is abnormal, there will be an affect on normal body activities causing hemorrhagic diseases. For example, if liver blood is deficient the following problems may appear: the symptoms of vertigo, contracture of spasm of muscles and tendons, impairment of flexion and extension of limbs or scanty menstruation and amenorrhea.

Promotion of Unrestrained Conditions for Qi

Liver *qi* possesses the function of regulation. It is responsible for the ascending, descending, and harmony of bodily *qi*. If the body's *qi* activity is harmonious and its ascending and descending are normal then the internal organs will continue their normal physiological activities. This function of the liver involves the following aspects:

1) The liver harmonizes the emotions. Traditional Chinese medicine considers that the normal or abnormal function of an unrestrained and free flowing *qi* is directly related to emotional activities, and that the mental state is not only dominated by the heart but also the liver. When *qi* activities are normal, the body has a harmonious circulation of *qi* and blood, an easy mind and happy emotions. If there is a dysfunction of *qi*'s free flow, it will directly affect the individual's emotional state. For example, liver *qi* stagnation will give rise to stuffiness and fullness of the chest, unhappy feelings, hypochondriasis, or even mental depression, crying, irregular menstruation, etc. If there is hyperactivity of the liver *qi*, there may be irritability, anger, insomnia, dream disturbed sleep, dizziness, vertigo, a ringing in the ear (tinnitus), or deafness. Any sudden change in the normal pattern of the emotions, especially great anger or mental depression, can affect the free flowing and spreading function of liver *qi* resulting in the pathological changes of liver *qi* stagnation.

2) Liver *qi* regulation can assist the ascending function of the spleen and the descending function of the stomach. This also involves bile secretion. Bile is necessary for the digestion of food and drink. If liver *qi* loses its harmonious flowing activities, it will affect the digestive function of the spleen and stomach and the excretion of bile, leading to the pathological symptoms of jaundice and bitter taste. It is very common that patients with stagnation of liver *qi* may not only have symptoms such as distension, pain in the chest and hypochondriac regions, anxiety, and anger, but also belching due to the failure of the stomach *qi* to descend and diarrhea caused by the dysfunctional ascending

34

of spleen *qi*. The former is known as "liver *qi* affecting the stomach," and the latter as "disharmonious conditions between the liver and the spleen."

Controlling the Tendons and the Luster
Reflected in the Nails

The tendons, fascia, and ligaments of the body all rely on the nourishment of liver blood. The movements of limbs and joints are not only the result of tendon flexing but are also related to the strength or weakness of liver blood. Only if liver blood is ample, can it nourish and supplement the tendons to continue the normal movements of the limbs. If the liver blood is insufficient and fails to nourish the tendons, the patient might experience symptoms such as tremors of the hands or feet, numbness of the limbs, or even difficulty in flexing and extending the limbs. If pathogenic heat exhausts the body fluid leading to the consumption of blood, then this will cause convulsion, opisthotonos and lockjaw (trismus). As the *Suwen* notes, "various kinds of wind diseases causing the eyes to stare upwards, twitching, dizziness, and vertigo, belong to the liver."[22]

It is said that, "Nails are the remains of the tendons,"[23] The dryness or moisture of the nails can reflect the sufficiency or insufficiency of liver blood. When liver blood is plentiful the tendons are supple and the nails appear hard and moist. If liver blood is insufficient and incapable of nourishing the tendons, then the nails may be thin, soft, brittle, and pale. The *Suwen* records, "The liver communicates with the tendons. The health of the liver is reflected in the luster of the nails."[24]

Opening into the Eye

The essential *qi* of the five *zang* and six *fu* organs flows upwards to nourish the eye. Thus those organs, especially the liver, have a close relationship with the eye. The liver's function of storing blood nourished the eye as its channel travels upwards connecting to the eye system. In the *Suwen* it says, "Liver *qi* is in communication with the eyes, so the eyes will be able to distinguish the five colors."[25] Thus an an abnormality of liver function can affect the eyes. If the liver blood is insufficient, there will be a dryness of the eyes, blurred vision, or night blindness. If pathogenic wind-heat attacks the liver channel, redness, swelling and pain in the eyes will be the symptoms. If the liver fire flares up, conjunctivitis may occur. If liver *yang* is in preponderance, dizziness and vertigo occur. Liver wind stirring up produces convulsions with the eyes staring upwards.

5.1. Kidneys

The main physiological functions and indicators of the kidneys are: 1) storing essence, controlling human reproduction, growth and development; 2) controlling water metabolism; 3) receiving *qi*; 4) producing marrow, filling up the brain, controlling the bones, manufacturing blood and influencing hair luster; 5) opening into the ear, perineal ante-tract and perineal post-tract; 6) connects with the urinary bladder to which it is connected from the exterior and the interior.

Storing Essence, Controlling Human Reproduction Growth and Development

Essence is defined as the basic substance both constituting the human body and maintaining its functional activities. As described in the *Suwen*, "Essence is the foundation of the human body."[26] Essence consists of two parts: congenital essence inherited from the parents and acquired essence transformed from food.

Essence is stored in the kidney and is known as kidney *qi*. It greatly influences the ability of reproduction, growth, and development. According to the *Suwen*:

At the age of fourteen, a woman will begin to menstruate. Her *ren* channel becomes unobstructed, and the *qi* of her *chong* channel is replete. This is why her menstruation becomes regular and she is able to conceive.... At the age of

36

forty-nine, a woman's *ren* channel becomes deficient, the *qi* of the *chong* channel becomes weakened and scanty, sexual energy becomes exhausted, and menstruation stops with the result that her body becomes old and she is no longer able to conceive.[27]

In reference to men, it continues:

As to a man.... At the age of sixteen, his kidney *qi* becomes even more abundant, he begins to have sexual energy and is full of semen that he can ejaculate. When he has sexual intercourse with a woman, he can cause conception.... At the age of fifty-six the liver *qi* begins to weaken, the tendons become inactive, sexual energy begins to run out, the semen becomes inadequate, the kidney becomes debilitated with the result that all parts of the body begin to grow old. At the age of sixty-four his hair and teeth are gone.[28]

Thus, according to traditional Chinese medicine, kidney *qi* plays an essential role in the function of reproduction, growth, and development. If this function is abnormal, infertility, infantile underdevelopment, maldevelopment, weakness of bone development, etc. will manifest.

Kidney essence is classified as *yin*, while *qi* is *yang*. Known as kidney *yin* and *yang*, they both restrict and depend on each other in order to maintain a dynamic physiological balance. If this balance is disrupted, pathological changes of hyperactivity or hypoactivity of kidney *yin* and *yang* will occur.

Clinically, a kidney *yin* deficiency may be manifested soreness, aching and weakness of the lumbar region and knees, blurred vision, poor memory, etc. A *yin* deficiency leading to *yang* preponderance will produce tidal fever, night sweating, dizziness, ringing in the ear (tinnitus), spermatorrhea, and sexual dreams. Kidney *yang* deficiency decreases the warming function of the kidney bringing on the symptoms of lassitude, coldness and pain in the lumbar region and the knees, cold extremities and frequent urination, leading to pathological conditions such as inadequate reproductive ability, impotence, premature ejaculation, and coldness of the uterus. If a certain degree of kidney *yin* or *yang* deficiency is reached then either may injure the other resulting in a loss of the body's dynamic physiological balance.

In addition, clinical manifestations such as frequent and clear urination, enuresis, incontinence of urine, spermatorrhea, premature ejaculation, etc. which show no heat or cold syndromes are considered to be a kidney *qi* deficiency. The clinical symptoms of dizziness, ringing in the ears, soreness and aching of the lumbar or knee region, infantile maldevelopment, etc., which demonstrate no clear cold or heat symptoms, are classified as kidney-essence deficiency.

Controlling Water Metabolism

The kidney plays an essential role in the distribution, regulation, and metabolism of water. As the *Suwen* says, "The kidney is the organ of water in charge of fluid."[29] Water is received by the stomach, transformed and transported by the spleen. Part of the fluid is sent down by the descending function of the lung until it finally reaches the kidney and is divided by the *qi* activity of the kidney *yang* into two parts: clear and turbid. The useful clear fluid is sent back up to the lung as *jin*, and the turbid waste fluid flows down into the urinary bladder to form urine, which is excreted. The distribution of water is related to the functions of the stomach, spleen, small intestine, large intestine, lung, urinary bladder, and *sanjiao*, but they all rely on the warming and pushing function of kidney *yang*. If kidney *yang* is insufficient, this may lead to retention of water resulting in scanty urination, retention of urine or frequent urination, enuresis, etc.

Receiving Qi

The reception of *qi* is controlled by the kidney, which leads it downward from the lung. If kidney *qi* is adequate, and its functioning normal, then breathing is even and smooth. In a deficient state, uneven breathing, dyspnea, and asthma exacerbated by exercise will occur.

Controlling Bones, Producing Marrow, and Influencing Hair Luster

Nourishment of the bone structure requires marrow, a product of kidney essence. The term "marrow" includes the bone marrow and the spinal cord. The brain is known as the "sea of marrow." Sufficiency of this essence produces a well developed and functioning skeletal system. Inadequate essence, however, may lead to a variety of syndromes: a sore, aching, and weak lumbar region and knees, weakness or atrophy of the lower limbs, infantile maldevelopment, delayed closing of the fontanelle, etc. Furthermore, according to traditional Chinese medicine, "teeth are the remainder of bone." Poor nourishment by kidney essence also causes looseness and loss of teeth.

Essence and blood generate each other. Ample essence makes sufficient blood. Hair is nourished by the blood and rooted on the basis of kidney *qi*. Therefore luster, moisture, dryness, roughness growth and falling out of hair is related to the sufficiency of kidney essence. As the *Suwen* says, "The kidney is in tune with the bones, its prosperity is reflected in the luster and moisture of the head hair."[30]

Opening into the Ear, Perineal Ante-Tract and Perineal Post-Tract

Auditory function is dependent on nourishment from the essential *qi* of the kidney. If that essence is sufficient, then keen hearing will result. Otherwise, there will be deafness and a ringing in the ears. The perineal ante-tract (including urethra and vagina) and post-tract (anus) have the action of reproduction and excretion through the function of kidney *qi*. Insufficiency will manifest as frequent urination, enuresis or scanty urine; for the reproductive organs there will be spermatorrhea, impotence, premature ejaculation, or infertility; bowel movements will be subject to either morning diarrhea or constipation.

5.2 Uterus

The uterine function is menstruation and foetal nourishment. It has a close relationship with the kidney, and the *chong* and *ren* channels. Normal menstruation, reproductive ability and optimum foetal nourishment follow sufficiency of *qi* and blood in the *chong* and *ren* channels. If their function is weak, then irregular menstruation, amenorrhea, and infertility will appear.

Section 2
The Six *Fu* Organs

1. Gall Bladder

The gall bladder is attached to the liver and stores bile. There is an ancient saying regarding the close relationship between the liver and bile, "The remaining *qi* of the liver flows to the gall bladder and turns into the juice of essence (bile)." Bile is continuously excreted into the intestinal lumen to assist in digestion. The bitter taste and yellow color of bile are significant in disease manifestations of bitter taste in the mouth, vomiting of bile, jaundice, etc. As the liver and the gall bladder are externally and internally related, the gall bladder is also involved in the free flow of *qi* concerning emotional activities.

Clinically, when some mental disorders or emotional symptoms such as fear and palpitation, insomnia, dream disturbed sleep, etc. occur, treatment can be applied by considering the gall bladder.

2. Stomach

Situated below the diaphragm, the stomach's upper outlet connects with the esophagus, and its lower outlet with the small intestine. Its main physiological function is to receive and digest food. The stomach is also known as the "sea of water and cereal." Food is digested here, then sent downward to the small intestine, where the essential substances are transformed and transported by the spleen to the whole body. The spleen and the stomach collectively are known as the "acquired foundation," that is, their proper nourishment establishes the foundation for a healthy life. Clinical diagnosis and treatment place great stress on the strength and weakness of the stomach and spleen *qi*. Generally, it is considered that whatever kind of disease occurs, if stomach *qi* is still strong, the prognosis will be good. It is said, "Stomach *qi* is the foundation of the human body. When there is stomach *qi*, there is life. When there is no stomach *qi* death will follow." Preserving stomach *qi* is therefore considered an important principle of treatment.

Normal stomach *qi* descends. If it fails to descend, symptoms such as anorexia, fullness, pain and distension of the upper abdomen, nausea, vomiting, hiccough, etc. will appear.

3. Small Intestine

The upper end of the small intestine connects with the stomach, its main function being to receive partially digested food from the stomach and further divide it into clear and turbid. The small intestine transfers the turbid residues to the large intestine. The spleen transports the clean essential substances to all parts of the body, and part of the water contained in food to the urinary bladder. Therefore, if diseased, the small intestine will not only affect the function of digestion and absorption, but also lead to urinary problems.

4. Large Intestine

The upper end of the large intestine is connected to the small intestine by the ileocecum, and its lower end connects to the anus. Its main physiological function is to receive the waste material sent down from the small intestine and, in the process of transporting it to the anus, absorb a part of its fluid, and convert it into feces to be excreted from the body. Dysfunction of the large intestine produces the symptoms of borborygmus and diarrhea; if the fluid is further exhausted, the symptoms will be constipation and so on.

5. Urinary Bladder

The main function of the urinary bladder is to store and discharge urine. It has an exterior and interior relationship with the kidney. Pathologically, if the urinary bladder has a dysfunction of *qi*, dysuria or retention of urine will appear. If its restrictive function is lost, there may be excessive urination or incontinence of urine.

6. *Sanjiao*

Sanjiao (three areas of the body cavity) is a general term for the three sections of the body trunk. The upper *jiao* contains the heart and lung, the middle *jiao* contains the spleen and stomach, and the lower *jiao* contains the kidney and urinary bladder. The following are the categories of function as described by the *Lingshu*:

> The function of the upper *jiao* is to act like a fog; the function of the middle *jiao* is maceration; the function of the lower *jiao* is to be an aqueduct.[31]

Thus the heart and lung function is to distribute *qi* and body fluid by a spreading and moistening action. The spleen and stomach must digest, absorb, and transfer the *qi*, blood, and body fluid transformed from the essential substances; a similar process to that of soaking in water to cause decomposition and dissolution. The kidney and urinary bladder function to transport fluids and water.

Pathological problems in any of the three *jiao* will effect the organs located there.

Chapter 3
Qi, Blood, and Body Fluid

Qi, blood, and body fluid are fundamental substances of the human body which sustain the normal physiological functions of the *zang-fu* organs and tissues.

Section 1
Qi

The character *qi* denotes a dynamic essence characterized by both substance and function. For example, clean *qi*, turbid *qi*, and the *qi* transformed from the essence of food are substantial *qi*, while the *qi* of the heart, liver, spleen, kidney, stomach, and the *qi* of the channels and collaterals are functional *qi*.

The classification of *qi* in the human body varies with its distribution, origin, and function.

1. Primary *Qi* (*yuan qi*)

Primary *qi* is the most important and fundamental *qi* originating from the congenital essence. It is nourished and replenished by the fundamental substance of food after birth. Primary *qi* is also known as the *qi* of the kidney, and is distributed to the whole body via the *sanjiao* functions. It arouses and promotes the activities of the *zang-fu* organs and tissues. If primary *qi* is congenitally deficient or exhausted due to chronic disease, then various pathological changes will occur.

2. Aggregative *Qi* (*zong qi*)

This is the combination of inhaled clean *qi* through the lung with the fundamental substance *qi* of food digested and absorbed by the stomach and spleen. Aggregative *qi* is accumulated in the chest and has the function of nourishing the lung and the heart, thus promoting respiration and blood circulation.

3. Nutrient *Qi* (*ying qi*)

Nutrient *qi* originates from the essential substance of food transformed by the spleen and stomach. It is the component part of blood flowing throughout the body. The *Suwen* states, "Nutrient *qi* is actually the essential *qi* transformed from food and water."[32] While in the *Lingshu* it is recorded:

> The nutrient *qi* is secreted by the body fluid, circulates in the blood vessels, and is transformed into blood to nourish the four extremities, the five *zang* and six *fu* organs.[33]

4. Defensive *Qi* (*wei qi*)

Defensive *qi* is mainly derived from the essential substances of food and water which form a part of the human body's *yang qi*. It circulates outside the vessels mainly spreading through the muscles and skin. Its physiological functions are 1) defending the body surface against the invasion of exogenous pathogenic factors, 2) warming and nourishing the tissues and organs, and 3) adjusting the opening and closing of the pores.

Section 2
Blood

Blood is transformed from the essence of food via the digestion and absorption of the spleen and stomach. According to the *Lingshu*, "When the middle *jiao* receives food and water, it transforms it into red fluid which is called blood."[34] After its formation, blood circulates incessantly throughout the body to nourish the *zang* and *fu* organs, the skin, the muscles, tendons, and bones in order to maintain their normal physiological activities.

Blood is the substantial basis for mental activities. Only when there the *qi* and blood are abundant can there be high spirits and clear minds. So in the *Suwen* it states, "Blood and *qi* are the spirits of man."[35] Pathological changes of blood cause symptoms of palpitation, insomnia, unconsciousness, delirium, etc.

Section 3
Body Fluid

Body fluid in traditional Chinese medicine is a general term for all normal liquid in the body including saliva, gastric fluid, intestinal fluid, joint cavity fluid, tears, nasal discharge, sweat, urine, etc.

Qi, Blood, and Body Fluid

Body fluid is derived from food and drink which is digested and absorbed by the spleen and stomach. It exists in the blood, tissues, and interstices of joints. A lucid and thin fluid termed *jin* fluid permeates the muscles and skin. Its main physiological function is to warm and nourish the muscles, and to moisten the skin. A turbid and viscous fluid called *ye* fluid supplies the joint cavities, brain, and body orifices. Its main physiological function is to lubricate the joints, tone the brain, and moisten the orifices. Although corresponding in general origin, formation, and function, *jin* and *ye* differ by their distribution, location, and individual functions. Since no definitive line can be drawn between the two, they are not clinically differentiated but are generally termed *jinye* (body fluid).

Chapter 4
The Theory of Channels and Collaterals

The theory of channels and collaterals is an important component of the theoretical system in traditional Chinese medicine. It covers the physiological functions and pathological changes of the channels and collaterals, their interrelations with the *zang-fu* organs, and is essential in guiding clinical practice, especially acupuncture treatment.

Section 1
The Formation and Functions of Channels and Collaterals

1. Channels and Collaterals System

The system of channels and collaterals constitutes the twelve regular channels, the eight extra channels, the fifteen collaterals, the twelve divergent channels, the musculo-tendinous and cutaneous regions of the twelve regular channels.

2. Channels and Collaterals Functions

1) Physiologically the channels and collaterals are considered to be a series of connecting passages through which *qi* and blood circulate to regulate the functions of the *zang-fu* organs, tissues, and sense organs. These passages also conduct the sensations and reactions (*deqi*) of acupuncture treatment.

The five *zang* and six *fu* organs, four limbs, nine orifices, skin, muscles, vessels, and tendons, although having their respective physiological functions, also maintain the harmonization and uniqueness of interior, exterior, upper, and lower parts of the body as a united and organic entity. This interconnection and organic combination relies upon the function of the channels and collaterals system.

All the tissues and organs of the human body need the nourishment of *qi* and blood in order to keep their normal physiological activities. The distribution and circulation of *qi* and blood throughout the body to nourish the *zang-fu*, tissues, and organs and to resist exogenous pathological factors depends on the transportation and conduction of the channels and collaterals. As the *Lingshu* records:

> The channels and collaterals are the passages through which blood and *qi* flow to nourish *yin* and *yang*, to moisten tendons and bones, and to lubricate the joints.[36]

2) Pathologically, channels and collaterals are the pathways through which the exogenous pathological factors are transmitted and their channels reflected. In the *Suwen* it is noted:

> When pathogenic factors invade the skin and the pores are open they enter the collaterals. When the collaterals become full, the pathogenic factors will move into the channels. When the channels are full, the pathogenic factors transmit to and reside in the *zang* and *fu* organs.[37]

The interior and exterior, upper and lower parts of the body form an integrated entity through the connecting network of channels and collaterals. So under pathological conditions every part of the body will affect the rest via the channels and collaterals. The channels and collaterals are not only the passages of disease transmission, but can also reflect pathological changes. Namely, the diseases of the *zang-fu* organs can be reflected on the body surface, especially in certain areas or at certain points, through the transmission of channels and collaterals.

3) In diagnosis, channels and collaterals have certain running courses that connect with the *zang-fu* organs. They also reflect pathological changes on the body surface. Therefore clinical diagnosis can be made according to symptoms that are related to those courses and their respective *zang-fu* organs.

4) In treatment, the theory of channels and collaterals is extensively used in clinical treatment for different branches of traditional Chinese medicine. Treatments using traditional medicinal herbs are based on their main actions vis-a-vis related *zang-fu* organs and channels. In the practice of acupuncture, the theory of channels and collaterals is the basis of all treatment and clinical practice. Point selection and prescription combinations are all made on this basis. By stimulating a certain point or area on the body surface the physiological functions of the channels and collaterals are aroused. This action is achieved by propagating sensation through the channels. Without this sensation it is hard to achieve a therapeutic effect.

Section 2
The Twelve Regular Channels

The twelve regular channels are a general term for the three *yin* and three *yang* channels of the hand and the three *yin* and three *yang* channels of the foot.

The Theory of Channels and Collaterals

1. The Lung Channel of the Hand Taiyin

The lung channel of the Hand Taiyin originates from the middle *jiao* and descends to connect with the large intestine (1). It turns around the upper orifice of the stomach (2), passing through the diaphragm (3) and enters the lung, forming part of the lung channels system (4). From the lung it flows upward to connect with the throat (5) and exits transversely from the arm pit (6). It then travels along the anterior-medial aspect of the upper arm (7), passing the cubital region and arrives at the Cunkou (8), the radial side of the wrist containing the radial artery for pulse palpation. Passing the thenar eminence (9), it travels along the radial border of the palm ending at the medial side of the tip of the thumb (Shaoshang, Lu. 11) (10). The branch separates from the Lieque (Lu. 7) (11) near to the wrist and goes directly to the radial side of the tip of the index finger (Shangyang, L.I. 1) (12) where it joins with the large intestine channels of the Hand-Yangming. (See *Fig.* 3)

Main pathological changes: Cough, asthma, hemoptysis, sore throat, pain and fullness of the chest, pain in the clavicular region, pain along the anterior-medial aspect of the arm, and shoulder pain.

2. The Large Intestine Channel of the Hang-Yangming

The large intestine channel of the Hang-Yangming starts from the tip of the index finger (Shangyang, L.I. 1) (1). Running upward along the radical aspect of the index finger, it passes through the inter-space of the first and second metacarpal bones, and ascends along the lateral anterior aspect of the upper arm to the highest point of the shoulder (2). It then travels along the anterior border of the acromion up to the seventh cervical vertebrae (3), then descends to the supraclavicular fossa (4) and enters the thoracic cavity to connect with the lung (5). It passes through the diaphragm (6) and enters the large intestine (7), forming part of the large intestine channel system.

The branch from the supraclavicular fossa travels upward to the neck (8) and to the cheek (9), and enters the lower teeth (10), then it curves around the upper lip and exits at the corner of the mouth (11), where it crosses the opposite large intestine channel of the Hand-Yangming at the philtrum (12). It ends at the side of the nose (Yingxiang, L.I. 20) (13) where it connects with the stomach channel of the Foot-Yangming. (See *Fig.* 4)

Main pathological changes: lower toothache, sore throat, epistaxis, runny nose, dryness of the mouth, swelling and pain of the neck, pain or motor impairment of the anterior-lateral aspect of the arm, etc.

3. The Stomach Channel of the Foot-Yangming

The stomach channel of the Foot-Yangming starts from the lateral side of the nose (Yingxiang, L.I. 20) (1). It flows upward to the bridge of the nose where it meets the urinary bladder channel of the Foot-Taiyang (Jingming, U.B. 1) (2). Turning downward along the lateral side of the nose, it enters the upper gum (3). Curving around the lips (4), it meets Chengjiang (Ren 24) at the mentolabial groove (5). Then it travels to the posterior aspect of the mandible passing through the Daying (ST. 5) (6) ascending in front of the ear and following the anterior hairline (7), it reaches the forehead (8).

The facial branch deviates from the anterior aspect of the Daying (St. 5) and runs downward to the Renying (St. 9) (9). It runs along the throat and enters the supraclavicular fossa (10). Going downward it passes through the diaphragm, enters the stomach (11), forming part of the stomach system, and connects with the spleen (12).

The straight line of the channels separates the supraclavicular fossa and runs downward along the middle mammillary line (13). It travels to the side of the umbilicus (2 *cun* lateral) (14)

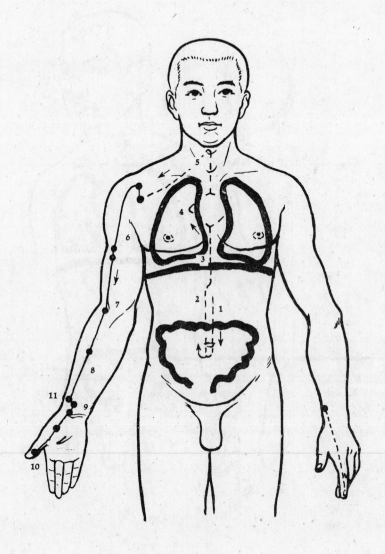

Fig. 3. The Lung Channel of the Hand Taiyin

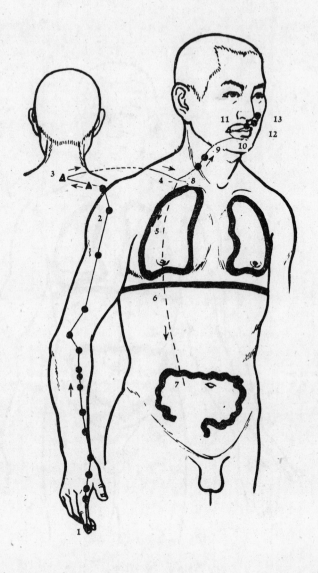

Fig. 4. The Large Intestine Channel
of the Hang-Yangming

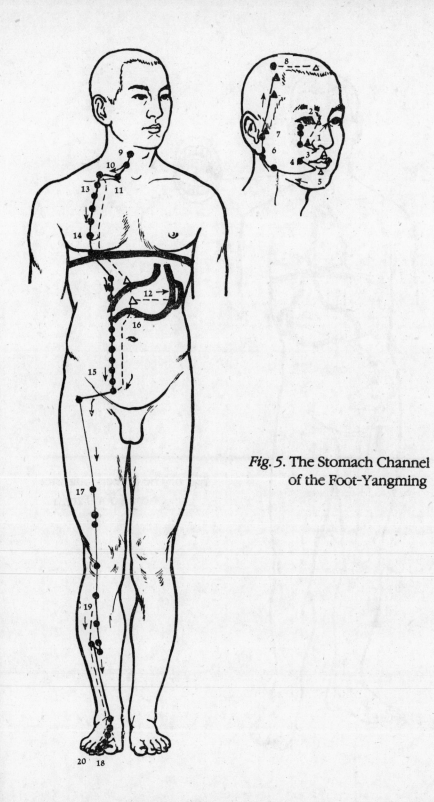

Fig. 5. The Stomach Channel
of the Foot-Yangming

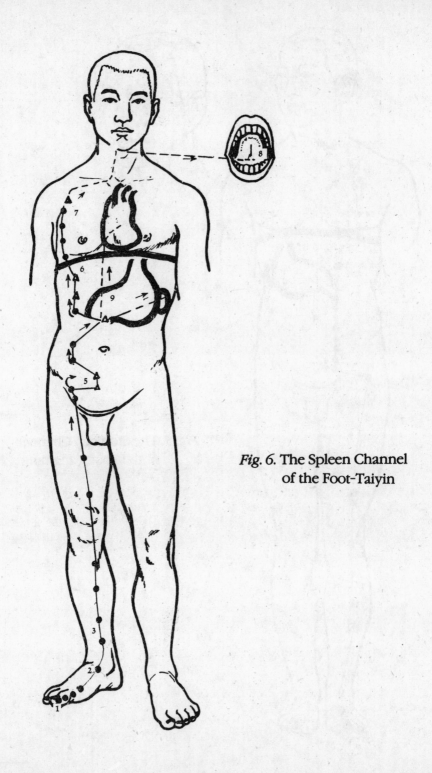

Fig. 6. The Spleen Channel
of the Foot-Taiyin

and descends to the inguinal groove, where it enters Pt. Qichong (St. 30) (15).[38]

The branch bifurcating from the lower orifice of the stomach (16) descends to the deep layer of the abdomen and joins the previous straight line of the channel at Pt. Qichong (St. 30) (15). Running downward it travels along the anterior aspect of the thigh and reaches the knee (17). From there it continues further down along the anterior border of the lateral aspect of the tibia to the dorsum of the foot and reaches the lateral side of the tip of the second toe (Lidui, St. 45) (18).

Another branch splits from Pt. Zusanli (St. 36) (19), and descends downward to enter the lateral side of the middle toe (20).

The branch from the dorsum of the foot parts from Chongyang (St. 42) (21) and flows anteriorly to the medial side of the tip of the great toe (Yinbai, Sp. 1) (22), where it communicates with the spleen channel of the Foot-Taiyin. (See *Fig.* 5)

Main pathological changes: borborygmus, abdominal distension, edema, stomach ache, vomiting, diabetes, deviated mouth and eyes, sore throat, epistaxis, high fever, perspiration, headache, mania, and pain along the course of the stomach channel.

4. The Spleen Channel of the Foot-Taiyin

The spleen of the Foot-Taiyin starts from the medial aspect of the tip of the big toe (Yinbai, Sp. 1) (1). It travels along the medial aspect of the foot at the junction between the red and white skin, ascends anteriorly to the medial malleolus (2) up to the medial aspect of the leg (3). It crosses and goes in front of the liver channel of the foot-Jueyin 8 *cun* above the medial malleolus. Passing through the anterior medial aspect of the thigh (4), it enters the abdomen (5) and the spleen (6), forming part of the spleen system, and connects with the stomach. From there it traverses the diaphragm (7), and runs alongside the esophagus. It arrives at the root of the tongue (8) and spreads over the lower surface of the tongue.

The branch goes from the stomach up through the diaphragm and flows into the heart (9) to join the heart channel of the Hand-Shaoyin. (See *Fig.* 6)

Main pathological changes: epigastric pain, abdominal distension, vomiting after eating food, belching, loose stools, jaundice, lassitude, heaviness of limbs, stiffness of the tongue, coldness, swelling and pain of the lateral side of the lower limb, motor impairment of the big toe, etc.

5. The Heart Channel of the Hand-Shaoyin

The heart channel of the Hand-Shaoyin commences at the heart (1) and pertains to the "heart system." It descends to pass through the diaphragm (2) and connects with the small intestine (3).

The ascending branch splits from the "heart system" up to the lung (4). Then it turns downward to the axilla (Jiquan, H. 1) (5). From there it goes along the posterior border of the medial aspect of the upper arm (6). Passing through the cubital region (7), it descends to the pisiform region proximal to the palm and enters the palm (8). Then it ends at the medial aspect of the tip of the little finger and links with the small intestine channel of the Hand-Taiyang. (See *Fig.* 7)

The branch splits from the "heart system" alongside the esophagus (9) to connect with the "eye system" (10).

Main pathological changes: Pain in the heart region, chest pains, sweating, heart palpitation, insomnia, dry throat, thirst, inner side arm pain, cold extremities, hot palms.

6. The Small Intestine Channel of the Hand-Taiyang

The small intestine channel of the Hand-Taiyang starts from the ulnar aspect of the tip of the little finger (Shaoże, S.I. 1) (1) and travels along the ulnar border of the hand dorsum upward to the posterior border of the lateral aspect of the upper arm (2). It passes through the cubital region curving around the scapular region (3) where it meets the *du* channel at Pt. Dazhui (Du. 14) (4). Then turning downward to the supraclavicular fossa (5), it connects with the heart (6). Alongside the esophagus, it passes through the diaphragm (7), reaches the stomach (8) and enters the small intestine (9) forming part of its channel system.

The branch separates from the supraclavicular fossa and ascends to the neck (10) and further up to the cheek (11). Going through the outer canthus, it turns into the ear (Tinggong, S.I. 19) (12).

Another branch deviates from the cheek. Running upward to the lower border of the infraorbital region, it reaches the inner canthus Pt. Jingming (U.B. 1) (13) to communicate with the urinary bladder channel of the Foot-Taiyang. (See *Fig.* 8)

Main pathological changes: Ringing in the ears, yellowish eye coloring, sore throat, swelling and pain under the jaw and in the neck, shoulder and upper external arm pain, abdominal pain and distension, frequent urination, etc.

7. The Urinary Bladder Channel of the Foot-Taiyang

The urinary bladder channel of the Foot-Taiyang originates from the inner canthus (Jingming, U.B. 1) (1). Passing through the forehead, it flows up to the vertex and meets the *du* channel at Pt. Baihui (Du. 20) (2).

A branch splits from the vertex and goes bilaterally down to the upper corner of the ear (3).

The straight line enters and connects with the brain from the vertex. It exits the brain at the neck region (4) and bifurcates into two lines. One line runs straight downward (1.5 *cun* lateral to the mid-line of the back) to the lumbar region (5), entering the body cavity to connect with the kidney and join with the urinary bladder (6), forming a part of its channel system. From there it descends along the posterior aspect of the thigh and ends in the popliteal fossa (7). Another line from the posterior aspect of the neck runs downward along the medial border of the scapula (3 *cun* lateral to the back mid-line) (8). Passing through the gluteal region (9), it meets the proceeding branch descending from the next region to the lumbar region in the popliteal fossa (10). From there it descends to the posterior aspect of the gastrocnemius muscle (11) and further to the lateral posterior side of the tip of the little toe (Zhiyin, U.B. 67) (12), where it communicates with the kidney channel of the Foot-Shaoyin. (See *Fig.* 9)

Main pathological changes: dysuria, enuresis, mania or depression, malaria, eye pains, lacrymation on exposure to the wind, nasal obstruction, runny nose, epistaxis, headache, stiffness of the neck, pain of the lower back and hip region and along the course of this channel on the posterior side of the leg.

8. The Kidney Channel of the Foot-Shaoyin

The kidney channel of the Foot-Shaoyin starts from the inferior aspect of the little toe (1), and runs obliquely towards the sole (Yongquan, K. 1) (2). Emerging from the lower aspect of the tuberosity of the navicular bone (3), it travels behind the medial malleolus and enters the heel (4). Ascending along the medial side of the leg (5), it passes the medial side of the popliteal fossa and goes further upward along the posterior-medial aspect of the thigh (6). Penetrating through the vertebral column of the lumbar region, it enters the kidney (7), forming part of its channel system, and links with the urinary bladder (8).

The straight line of the channel comes out from the kidney. It ascends passing through the liver (9) and diaphragm (10), enters the lung (11), and runs alongside the throat (12), ending at the root of the tongue.

A branch springs from the lung, links with the heart (13), and flows into the chest to communicate with the pericardium

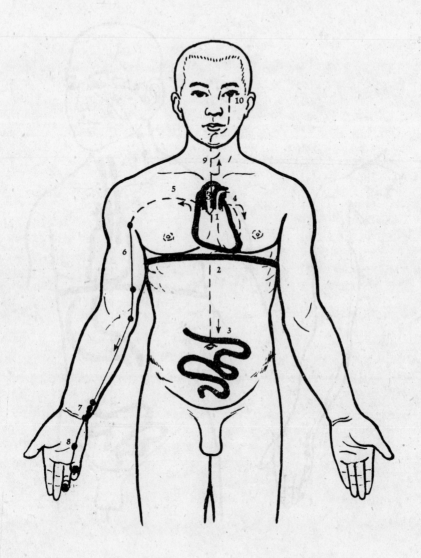

Fig. 7. The Heart Channel of the Hand-Shaoyin

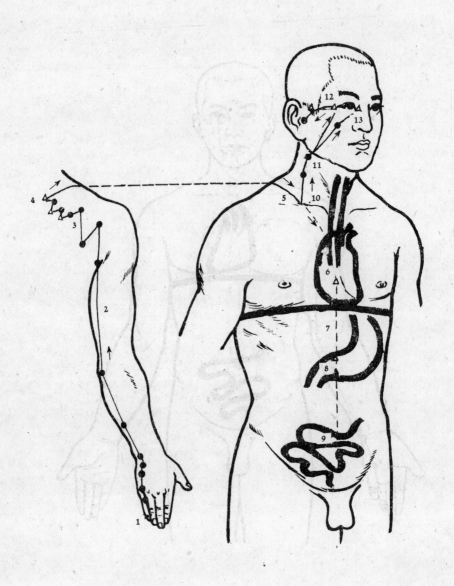

Fig. 8. The Small Intestine Channel of the Hand-Taiyang

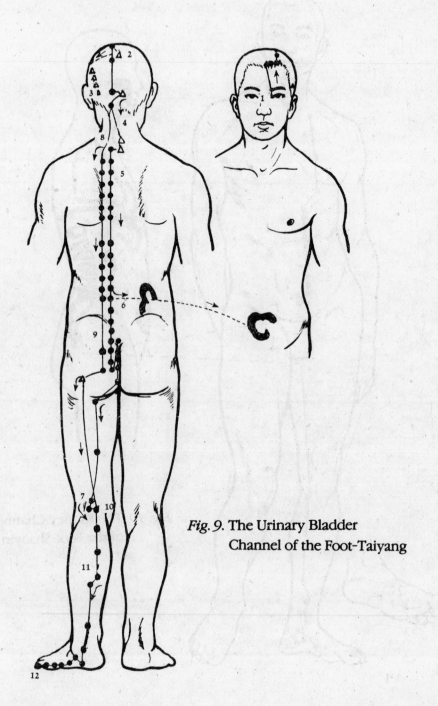

Fig. 9. The Urinary Bladder
Channel of the Foot-Taiyang

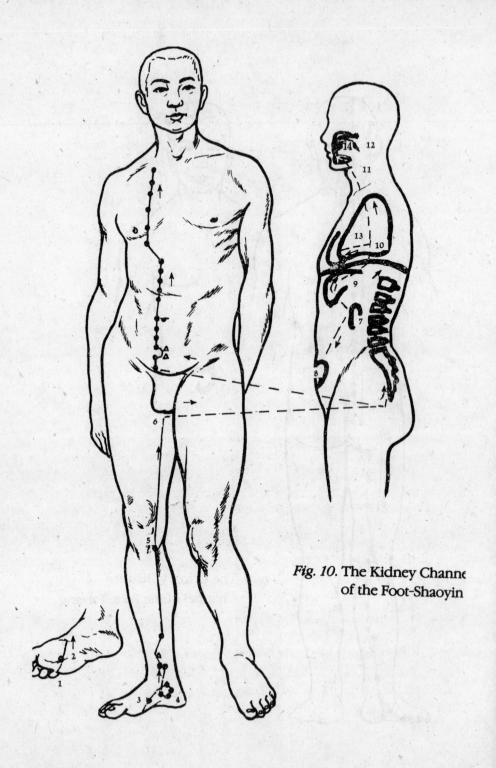

Fig. 10. The Kidney Channel of the Foot-Shaoyin

channel of the Hand-Jueyin. (See *Fig.* 10)

Main pathological changes: shortness of breath, dyspnea, cough, hemoptysis, dizziness, vertigo, dryness of the tongue, sore throat, low back pain, frequent urination, enuresis, spermatorrhea, impotence, dysuria, constipation or diarrhea, irregular menstruation, pain of the lumbar spine or along the posterior-medial side of the thigh, weakness of the lower limbs, feverish sensation of palms and soles, etc.

9. The Pericardium Channel of the Hand-Jueyin

The pericardium channel of the Hand-Jueyin originates in the chest (1). It enters the pericardium, then descends to pass through the diaphragm (2). Running through the abdomen, it connects successively with the upper, middle, and lower *jiao*.

A branch springs from the chest (1) and emerges from the costal region to a point 3 *cun* below the anterior axillary fold (Tianchi, P. 1) (3). It then ascends to the axillary fossa and along the medial aspect of the upper arm (4), it runs downward between the lung channel of the Hand-Taiyin and the heart channel of the Hand-Shaoyin (5). After emerging in the cubital fossa, it goes further downward to the forearm between the tendons of the m. palmaris longus and m. flexor carpi radialis (6). It enters the palm (7) and passes along the middle finger to its tip (Zhongchong, P. 9) (8).

Another branch splits from the palm at Pt. Laogong (P. 8) (9), runs along the ring finger to its tip (10) (Quanchong, S.J. 1) and communicates with the *sanjiao* channel of the Hand-Shaoyang. (See *Fig.* 11)

Main pathological changes: palpitation, irritability, pain in the precardiac region, stuffy chest, mental disorder, swelling and pain of the axillary region, spasm or contracture of the elbow, feverish sensation in the palm, etc.

10. The *Sanjiao* Channel of the Hand-Shaoyang

The *sanjiao* channel of the Hand-Shaoyang originates from the tip of the ring finger (Guanchong, S.J. 1) (1). It travels upward between the fourth and fifth metacarpal bones and along the dorsal side of the wrist and the lateral side of the forearm between the radius and ulna, it passes through the olecranon (2). Then it runs along the lateral aspect of the upper arm and reaches the shoulder region (3) where it travels across and behind the gall bladder channel of the Foot-Shaoyang. Crossing over the shoulder, it enters the supraclavicular fossa (4) and spreads in the chest to connect with the pericardium (5). It then proceeds through the diaphragm (6) down the abdomen, and communicates with the upper, middle, and lower *jiao* forming a part of the *sanjiao* channel system.

A branch springs from the chest (7) and runs upward exiting from the supraclavicular fossa, and ascends to the neck (8). Running along the posterior border of the ear (9), it crosses from the superior aspect of the ear to the corner of the forehead (10). Then it turns downward to the cheek and·terminates in the infraorbital region (11).

Another branch arises from the anterior aspect of the ear (12). It crosses the former branch at the cheek and reaches the outer canthus (13) to link with the gall bladder channel of the Foot-Shaoyang. (See *Fig.* 12)

Main pathological changes: deafness, ringing in the ears, sore throat, pain of the outer canthus, swelling of the cheek, pain of the retroauricular region, shoulder and lateral aspects of the upper arm and elbow, dysuria, edema, enuresis, abdominal distension, etc.

11. The Gall Bladder Channel of the Foot-Shaoyang

The gall bladder channel of the Foot-Shaoyang starts from the outer canthus (Tongziliao, G.B. 1) (1) and ascends to the corner of the forehead (Hånyan, G.B. 4) (2) and then winds downward to the retroauricular region (Fengchi, G.B., 20) (3). It then runs along the lateral side of the neck emerging in front of the *sanjiao* channel of the Hand-Shaoyang (4). It traverses behind the *sanjiao* channel of the Hand-Shaoyang at the shoulder region and travels further down to the supraclavicular fossa (5).

The retroauricular branch passes through the ear (6) and emerges in front of the ear at the posterior side of the outer canthus (7). A branch comes out from the outer canthus (8), runs downward to the Daying (St. 5) (9) and meets the *sanjiao* channel of the Hand-Shaoyang at the infraorbital region (10). Descending and passing through the Jiache (St. 6) (11), it reaches to the neck and enters the supraorbital fossa to meet with the main line of the channel (12). From there it further descends and enters the chest (13), passes through the diaphragm to connect with the liver (14) and enters the gall bladder (15), forming part of its channel system. It then travels interiorly in the hypochondriac region, emerging at the lateral side of the lower abdomen near the femoral artery in the inguinal region (16). Then it curves along the margin of the public hair and runs transversely into the hip region (Huantiao, G.B. 30) (17).

The straight line of the channel travels downward from the supraclavicular fossa (18), and further down to the axillary region (19). Along the lateral side of the chest (20) and through the free ends of the floating ribs (21), it meets the former branch at the hip region (22). It then travels downward along the lateral side of thigh to the lateral side of the knee (23). Further descending along the anterior aspect of the fibula (24), it reaches the lower end of the fibula, and the anterior aspect of the lateral malleolus (25). Following the dorsum of the foot, it terminates at the lateral side of the fourth toe's tip (Foot-Qiaoyin, G.B. 44) (26).

The branch splitting from Foot-Linqi (G.B. 41) (27) runs between the 1st and 2nd metatarsal bones to the hairy area of the big toe (Dadun, Liv. 1) (28) where it communicates with the liver channel of the Foot-Jueyin. (See *Fig.* 13)

Main pathological changes: alternate chills and fever, bitter taste in the mouth, blurred vision, vertigo, hypochondriac pain, migraine, pain in the supraclavicular fossa, pain of the outer canthus and axillary fossa, malaria, pain along the lateral side of the thigh, knee and leg, pain and motor impairment of the fourth toe, etc.

12. The Liver Channel of the Foot-Jueyin

The liver channel of the Foot-Jueyin originates from the dorsal hairy region of the big toe (Dadun, Liv. 1) (1). Ascending along the dorsum of the foot, it flows further upward to the anterior aspect of the medial malleolus (2) where it crosses behind the spleen channel of the Foot-Taiyin to the area 8 *cun* above the medial malleolus (3). Then it runs upward to the medial side of the knee (4) and along the medial aspect of the thigh (5) into the public hair region (6). From there it curves around the external genitalia and travels up to the lower abdomen (7). Alongside the stomach, it enters the liver (6), forming part of its channel system, and connects with the gall bladder (9). Then it proceeds upward to pass through the diaphragm (10) and disperses in the costal and hypochondriac region (11). Ascending along the posterior aspect of the throat (12), it emerges in the nasopharynx region (12) to connect with the "eye system" (13). Extending further upward, it exits from the forehead (14) and meets the Du channel at the vertex (15).

A branch arising from the "eye system" descends to the cheek (16) and curves around the internal surface of the lips (17). another branch separating from the liver (18), passes through the diaphragm and enters the lung (19) to link with the lung channel of the Hand-Taiyin. (See *Fig.* 14)

Main pathological changes: pain and distension of the hypochondrium, stuffiness of the chest, vomiting, diarrhea, vertex headache, hernia, dysuria, enuresis, pain and distension of the

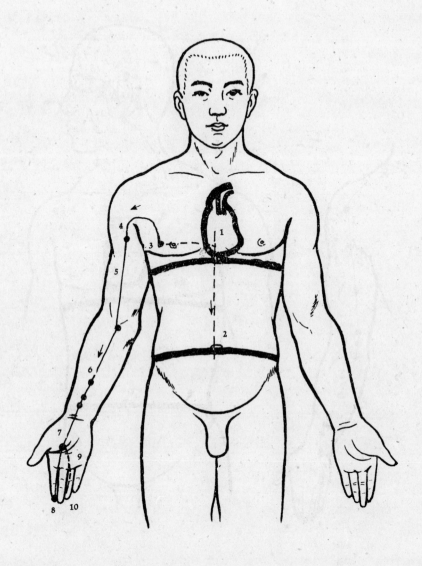

Fig. 11. The Pericardium Channel of the Hand-Jueyin

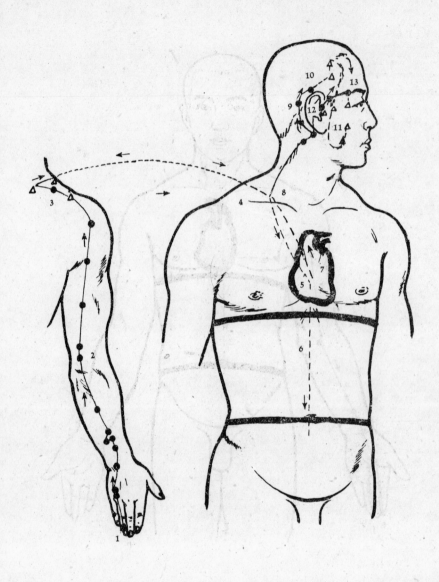

Fig. 12. the Sanjiao Channel of the Hand-Shaoyang

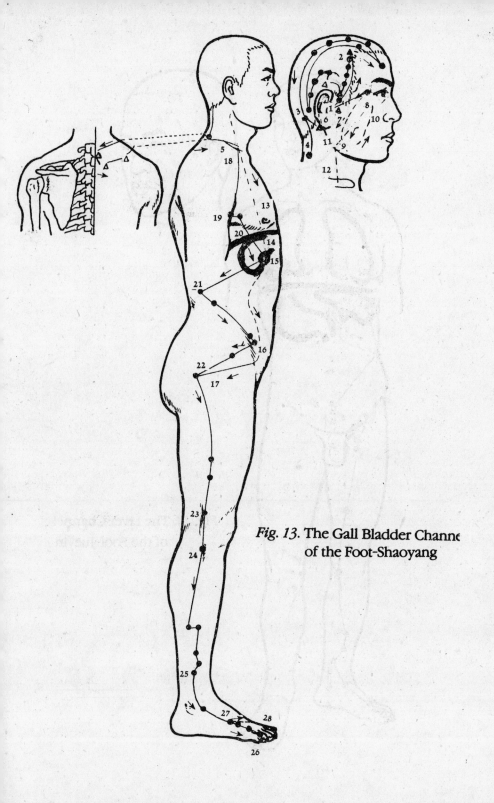

Fig. 13. The Gall Bladder Channel
of the Foot-Shaoyang

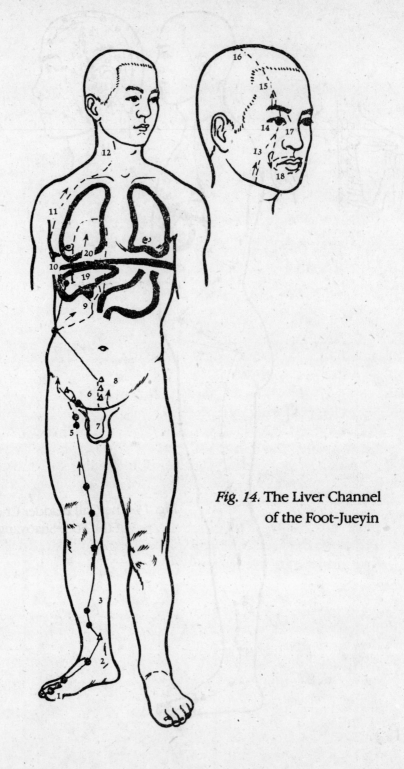

Fig. 14. The Liver Channel
of the Foot-Jueyin

lateral lower abdomen, lumbago, irregular menstruation, mental disorders, etc..

Section 3
Pathways, Conjunctures, Exterior-Interior Relationships and the Order of *Qi* Flow in the Channels

1. Pathways and Conjunctures

The running direction and the interconjunction of the twelve regular channels compose the following network: the three *yin* channels of the hand run from the chest to the hand, connecting with the three *yang* channels of the hand; the three *yang* channels of the hand run from the hand to the head, joining with the three *yang* channels of the foot; the three *yang* channels of the foot travel from the head to the foot, uniting the three *yin* channels of the foot; the three *yin* channels of the foot proceed from the foot up to the abdomen, linking with the three *yin* channels of the hand.

2. Exterior-Interior Relationships and the Order of the *Qi* Flow in the Channels

The twelve regular channels of the hand *yin-yang* and foot *yin-yang* respectively have a connecting relationship with their pertaining *zang* or *fu* organ. Specifically, *yin* channels pertain to *zang* organs and connect with *fu* organs, while *yang* channels pertain to *fu* organs and connect with *zang* organs. The exterior-interior relationship of the twelve regular channels is the same as the exterior-interior relationship of the *zang* and *fu* organs.

Table 2.

Schematic Diagram of Qi Flow Order in The Twelve Regular Channels

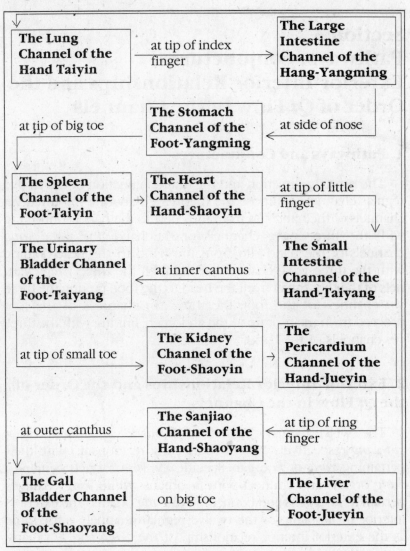

Channels which have an exterior-interior relationship run opposite each other on the lateral and medial aspects of the four limbs (except the liver channel of the Foot-Jueyin and the spleen channel of the Foot-Taiyin which change their position 8 *cun* above the medial malleolus of the lower limbs). These channels then connect with each other on the hand or foot, forming the six pairs of exteriorly-interiorly related channels of the *zang-fu* organs. *Qi* flows continually, circulating throughout the channels in the following manner as shown in *Table 2*.

Section 4
Eight Extra Channels

The eight extra channels are the following group of eight channels: Ren, Du, Chong, Dai, Yinwei, Yangwei, Yinqiao, and Yangqiao. They differ from the twelve regular channels in that they neither pertain to any *zang* or *fu* organ, nor do they share an exterior-interior relationship between each other. Their main function is to regulate the circulation of *qi* and blood in the twelve regular channels. When these regular channels are overfull, excess *qi* and blood flow into the eight extra channels to be stored for later use.

1. The Ren Channel

The Ren channel connects with all the *yin* channels of the body and is therefore known as the "sea of *yin* channels." In women, it is responsible for pregnancy and foetal nourishment.

The Ren channel commences within the lower abdomen and exits at the perineum (1). It ascends anteriorly to the public region (2). Along the internal abdomen, it flows upward to pass through Pt. Guanyuan (Ren 4) and other points, and reaches the throat (3). Flowing further upward, it curves around the lips (4),

Fig. 15. The Ren Channel

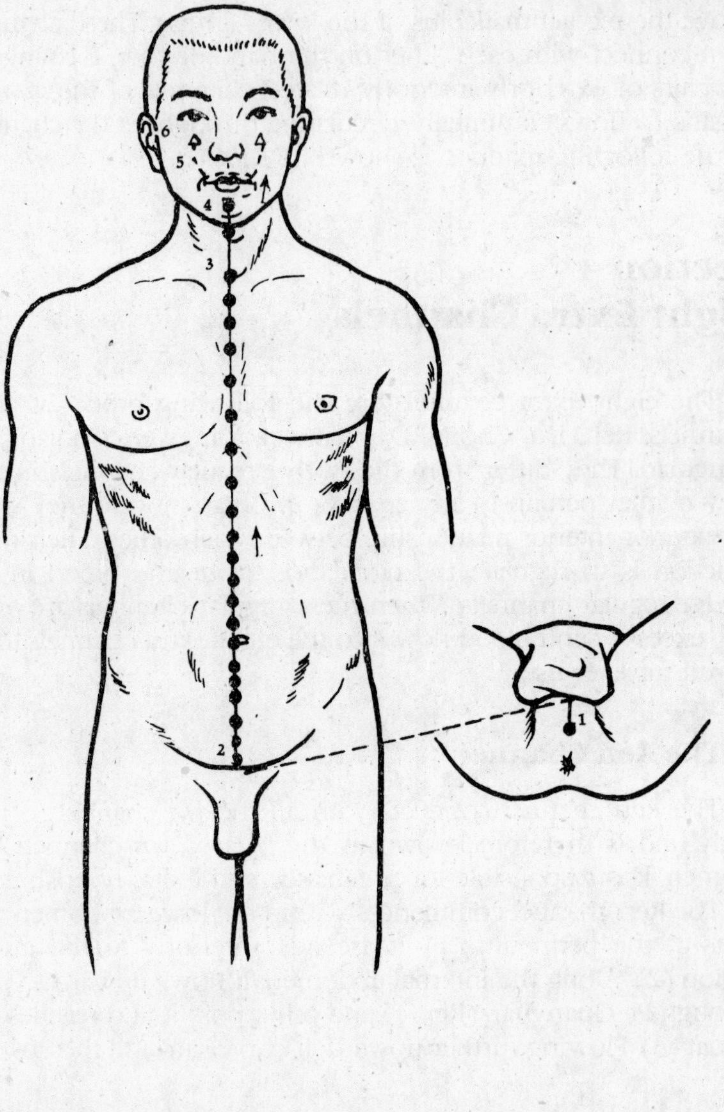

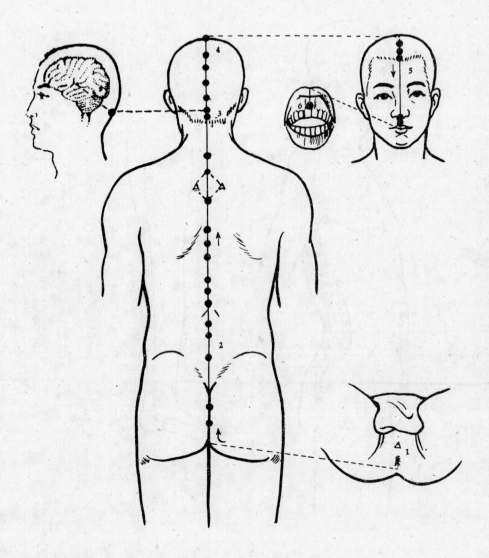

Fig. 16. The Du Channel

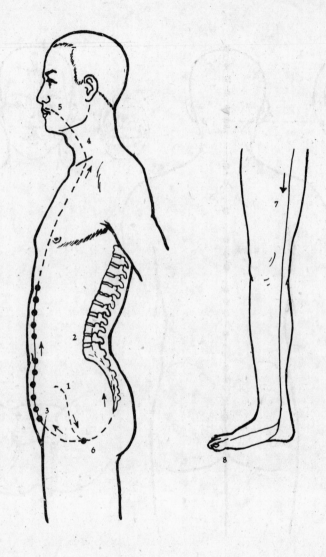

Fig. 17. The Chong Channel

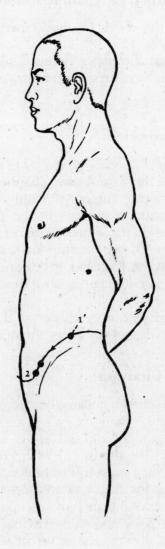

Fig. 18. The Dai Channel

passes through the cheek (5), and emerges in the infraorbital region (6). (See *Fig.* 15)

Main pathological changes: hernia, leukorrhea, lumps in the lateral lower abdomen, irregular menstruation, abortion, infertility, etc.

2. The Du Channel

The Du channel governs all the *yang* channels of the body, so it is known as the "sea of *yang* channels."

The Du channel commences within the lower abdomen. Traveling downward, it appears in the perineum (1). It then flows upward inside the spinal column (2) to the nape of the neck (Fengfu, Du 16) (3), entering the brain and ascends to the vertex (4). Along the forehead, it descends to the nose bridge, then to the lips (5), entering the labial frenulum inside the upper lip (6). (See *Fig.* 16)

Main pathological changes: stiffness of the spine, opisthotonos, pain of the back, mental disorders, infantile convulsion, etc.

3. The Chong Channel

The Chong channel regulates the circulation of *qi* and blood of the twelve regular channels, so it is known as the "sea of the twelve regular channels" and the "sea of blood."

It originates in the uterus (1) where three branches immediately arise. The first branch travels along the posterior wall of the abdominal cavity, then ascends and runs inside the spinal column (2). The second branch travels up to the umbilicus along the anterior wall of the abdominal cavity (3) and spreads in the chest, then flows upward to the throat (4) and circles around the lips (5). The third branch descends and emerges in the perineum (6), and runs downward along the medial aspect of the thigh (7), terminating at the big toe (8). (See *Fig.* 17)

Main pathological changes: irregular menstruation, amenorrhea, uterine bleeding, deficient lactation, hematemesis, etc.

4. The Dai Channel

The Dai channel possesses the function of binding and restricting other channels. It starts below the hypochondriac region (1), runs obliquely downward, then transversely around the waist like a belt (2). (See *Fig.* 18)

Main pathological changes: abdominal distension and coldness of the lumbar region, like "sitting in water."

5. The Yinwei Channel

The Yinwei channel binds the six *yin* channels together and joins with the Ren channel.

Commencing from the medial aspect of the lower leg (1), it runs along the medial aspect of the thigh (2) up to the abdomen (3) to meet with the Foot-Taiyin channel. It then passes through the chest (4) and communicates with the Ren channel at the neck region (5). (See *Fig.* 19)

Main pathological changes: heart pain, mental depression, etc.

6. The Yangwei Channel

The Yangwei channel connects with the six *yang* channels and communicates with the Du channel.

It originates at the lateral side of the heel (1). Running upward to the external malleolus (2), it ascends along the gall bladder channel of the Foot-Shaoyang up to the hip region (3). Passing through the posterior aspect of the hypochondriac (4), axillary, shoulder and neck regions (5), it further travels upward to the cheeks (6) and forehead (7), then turns backward to the back of the neck, where it meets with the Du channel (8). (See *Fig.* 20)

Main pathological changes: alternate chills and fever, low back pain, etc.

7. The Yinqiao Channel

The Yinqiao channel has the function of controlling the movements of the lower limbs and eyelids.

It starts from the posterior aspect of the navicular bone (1), and ascends to the anterior aspect of the medial malleolus (2). Running along the medial aspect of the thigh (30, to the external genitalia (4), it ascends further along the medial aspect of the chest (5) to the supraclavicular fossa (6). It then passes through the anterior aspect of Pt. Renying (St. 9) (7) up to the zygoma (8), and reaches the inner canthus to communicate with the *yangqiao* channel (9) and Foot-Taiyang channel. (See *Fig.* 21)

Main pathological changes: inward splay-foot, sore throat, hypersomnia, retention of urine, etc.

8. The Yangqiao Channel

The Yangqiao channel regulates the movements of the lower limbs and eyelids.

It starts from the lateral side of the heel (1). Ascending along the lateral malleolus, it passes the posterior border of the fibula. Then it runs upward along the lateral aspect of the thigh to the abdomen and the lateral aspect of the hypochondriac region, where it winds over the shoulder (2), passes through the neck to the corner of the mouth (3) and enters into the inner canthus to meet with the Yinqiao channel. It runs further upward along the urinary bladder channel of the Foot-Taiyang to the forehead and communicates with the gall bladder channel of the Foot-Shaoyang at the nape of the neck (4). (See *Fig.* 22)

Main pathological changes: outward splay-foot, insomnia, pain in the inner canthus, etc.

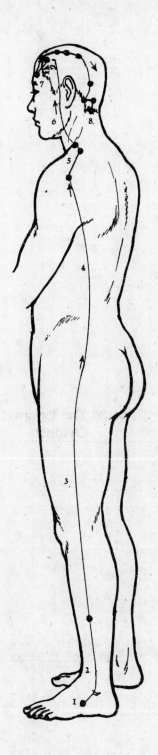

Fig. 19. The Yinwei
Channel

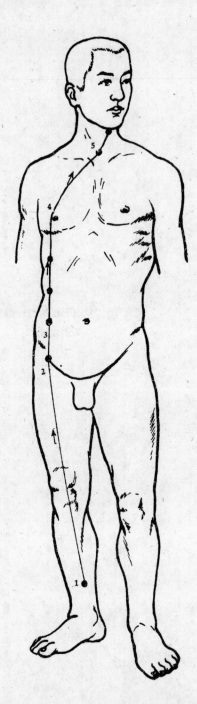

Fig. 20. The Yangwei
Channel

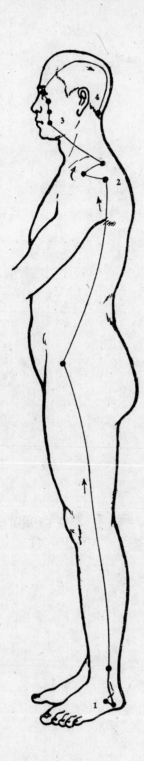

Fig. 21. The Yinqiao
Channel

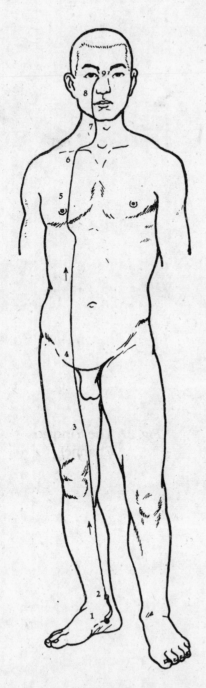

Fig. 22. The Yangqiao
Channel

Section 5
The Fifteen Collaterals

The collaterals are the transverse branches which bifurcate from the channels. There are fifteen collaterals in all, that is, each of the twelve regular channels has a collateral, plus the Ren and Du channels, and the great collateral of the spleen.

These collaterals are distributed in certain areas of the body. On the four limbs, the collaterals of the *yin* channels run towards the *yang* channels which are exteriorly-interiorly related; while the collaterals of the *yang* channels run to their exteriorly-interiorly related *yin* channels. On the trunk, the collateral of the Ren channel spreads over the abdomen. The collateral of the Du channel disperses throughout the head and branches off to join the Taiyang channel of the foot. The great collateral of the spleen is distributed over the chest and hypochondriac regions.

The collaterals strengthen the function of the twelve regular channels and closely connect the exterior-interior related channels. They also assist the transportation and distribution of *qi* and blood in order to moisten and nourish the whole body (see *Table* 3).

Section 6
The Twelve Divergent Channels

The twelve regular channels have certain courses internally pertaining to the *zang-fu* organs and externally to the connecting joints and limbs. Each channel also has a deviating or diverging branch penetrating the body cavity which is termed a divergent channel.

The divergents of *yang* channels run up from the limbs and enter into the internal organs of the chest and abdominal

Table 3

Distribution of the Fifteen Collaterals

Collateral	Acu-point	Location	Connection
Hand Taiyin	Lieque (Lu.7)	0.5 cun above wrist	Hand Yangming
Hand Shaoyin	Tongli (H.5)	1 cun above wrist	Hand Taiyang
Hand Jueyin	Neiguan (P.6)	2 cun above wrist	Hand Shaoyang
Hand Yangming	Painli (L.I.6)	3 cun above wrist	Hand Taiyin
Hand Taiyang	Zhizheng (S.I.7)	5 cun above wrist	Hand Shaoyin
Hand Shaoyang	Waiguan (S.J.5)	2 cun above wrist	Hand Jueyin
Foot Yangming	Fenglong (St.40)	8 cun above malleolus	Foot Taiyin
Foot Taiyang	Feiyang (U.B.58)	7 cun above malleolus	Foot Shaoyin
Foot Shaoyang	Guangming (G.B.37)	5 cun above malleolus	Foot Jueyin
Foot Taiyin	Gongsun (Sp.4)	1 cun proximal to phalangeal joint of big toe	Foot Yangming
Foot Shaoyin	Taichong (Liv.3)	Posterior to malleolus on heel	Foot Taiyang
Foot Jueyin	Ligou (Liv.5)	5 cun above malleolus	Foot Shaoyang
Ren Channel	Wuyi (St.15)	Below xyphoid process	Over abdomen
Du Channel	Changqiang (Du.1)	At tip of coccyx	Over the head through spine
Great Collateral of Spleen	Dabao (Sp.21)	3 cun below auxillary fossa	Over chest & hypochondriac region

regions. Most of them again emerge from the nape of the neck and rejoin the *yang* regular channels from whence they originally branched. The divergents of the *yin* regular channels separate from their primary channels and travel parallel to meet with and rejoin the *yang* channels to which they have an exterior-interior relationship. Among these twelve divergent channels, no matter whether *yin* or *yang*, all start their deviation from the the area above the knee or elbow and finally reunite only with the six *yang* channels. Internally, both *yin* and *yang* divergents enter the chest and abdomen to associate with the pertaining *zang* or *fu* organs to which their parent regular channel has an exterior-interior relationship. In addition, the divergent channels of the three foot *yang* regular channels pass through the heart and travel up to the head region. The divergent channels of the three hand *yang* regular channels penetrate through to the internal organs from the axillary fossa, and proceed through the throat, to arrive at the head and facial regions.

The main function of the twelve divergent channels is to strengthen the exterior-interior relationship of the twelve regular channels and so form closer ties between all parts of the body.

Section 7
The Twelve Musculotendinous Regions of the Regular Channels

The musculotendinous regions of the twelve regular channels are the continuation of this channel system extending over the extremities of the organic body. the feature of their distribution is that they run on the body surface and do not enter the internal organs. Their traveling courses start from the extremities of the four limbs and proceed to the head and trunk. Taiyang and

Shaoyin run to the posterior aspect, Shaoyang and Jueyin to the lateral side, and Yangming and Taiyin to the anterior aspect. All the musculotendinous regions of the regular channels are interconnected with each other.

Their main physiological function is to restrict the bones and facilitate the joints. As the *Suwen* records, "The musculotendinous regions of the regular channels are in charge of the bones and facilitate the joints."[39]

Section 8
The Twelve Cutaneous Regions of the Regular Channels

The twelve cutaneous regions indicate the superficial range of the twelve regular channels on the body surface. As the *Suwen* describes, "The skin region belongs to the system of regular channels."[40]

The cutaneous regions are closely associated with the internal organs. Therefore, exogenous pathogenic factors can gradually be transmitted to and invade the internal organs through the cutaneous regions. Conversely, the diseases of the *zang-fu* organs can be reflected on the cutaneous regions of the body surfaces. This theory of cutaneous regions has a practical value for the application of diagnosis and treatment in traditional Chinese medicine.

Chapter 5
Etiology

Traditional Chinese medicine posits a uniquely relative relationship between the *zang-fu* organs and tissues of the human body, as well as between the human body and the natural environment. All are in a relatively balanced state in order to maintain the body's normal physiological function. When this balance is destroyed disease results.

Through long term clinical practice, the ancient Chinese realized that there are many factors which may bring about imbalances in the human body and thus disease; climate abnormalities, pestilence, emotional stimulation, injury by irregular diet or overstrain, trauma, insect-bites, etc., plus pathological products of disease outcome, such as blood stasis, phlegm-humor, etc. All of these contribute to imbalances within the human system.

The etiology of traditional Chinese medicine uses clinical manifestations as evidence, i.e., through the analysis of symptoms and signs of a disease, one can find its causative factors. This is technically termed "checking syndromes to find causative factors of a disease." For our study of etiology, we must concern ourselves with the properties of pathogenic factors and the characteristics of how and why they cause disease.

Traditional Chinese medicine holds that the occurrence of a disease not only depends on exogenous factors, but more importantly is decided by body resistance. Chinese medicine terms all exogenous pathogenic factors as *xie qi*, while the body's resistance against disease is termed *zheng qi*. When the *zheng qi* is relatively weak, *xie qi* will have an opportunity to attack and upset the body's *yin-yang* balance; this leads to disease. The *Suwen* records, "If a pathogenic factor attacks the body, then the *zheng qi* must be weak."[41] Furthermore, "When *zheng qi* exists in the interior, the pathogenic factor will be unable to interfere."[42] Therefore the invasion of *xie qi* is due to the insufficiency of *zheng qi*, this is the root cause. *Xie qi* is necessary condition for the occurrence of a disease. The development, transformation, and prognosis of a disease depend on the forced balance of *zheng qi* and *xie qi*.

Section 1
Six Exogenous Factors

Spring-wind, summer-heat, summer-fire, late summer-dampness, autumn-dryness, and winter-cold are the six variations in the climate of the four seasons. They are also known as the "six climatic factors" or the "six exogenous *qi*."

The human body has the ability to adapt to climatic variations. However, when bodily resistance is too low to adapt to climatic changes or if there is an abnormal altering of the weather which surpasses the body's adaptability, then the six climatic *qi* will become pathogenic factors bringing about the occurrence of disease. Therefore the climatic *qi* are all considered to be exogenous pathogenic factors.

Diseases which are not caused by exogenous pathogenic factors, but have symptoms similar to the syndromes of wind, cold, summer-heat, dampness, and dryness are termed internal heat, internal damp, internal dryness, and internal fire. These endogenous pathogenic factors are the outcome of dysfunctions of the *zang* and *fu* organs.

1. Wind

Pathogenic wind prevails in spring and is a common pathogenic factor of the common cold. It causes diseases together with other pathogenic factors, e.g., wind-cold, wind-heat, wind-damp, etc.

1) Wind is a *yang* pathogenic factor, characterized by upward flowing. When it attacks the human body, it often affects the upper region first.[43] For example, if exogenous pathogenic wind causes a common cold, its symptoms are headache, nasal obstruction, itching or sore throat, etc., which are confined to the upper body. If pathogenic wind together with dampness induces disease the symptoms are swelling of the eyes and face.

2) Wind is characterized by outward dispersion. If pathogenic wind attacks the body, it may affect the defensive *qi* causing derangement in the opening and closing of pores. The clinical symptoms are fever, sweating, aversion to wind, etc.

3) Wind blows in gusts and is characterized by rapid change. In the *Suwen* it says, "The wind is good at traveling and undergoes change frequently."[44] Diseases caused by wind are marked by migrating disease location and symptoms that appear and disappear. Onset is abrupt and disappearance hasty, e.g., migrating joint pain of *bi* syndromes, which usually involve joint pains, and intolerable itching of urticaria.

4) Wind is characterized by constant moving. Pathogenic wind causes motor impairment or abnormal motion of the trunk

or limbs manifested by convulsion, opisthotonos, spasm, and tremor of the four limbs, and rigidity of the neck. In the *Suwen* it says, "Predominant wind causes symptoms characterized by movements."[45]

5) Wind is liable to associate itself with other pathogenic factors. Pathogenic wind is apt to be accompanied with cold, damp, or heat to become wind-cold, wind-damp, or wind-heat pathogenic factors.

Wind may be also associated with some pathological products such as phlegm, forming pathogenic wind-phlegm. The commonly seen symptoms caused by exogenous pathogenic wind are known as *shangfeng* (wind damage).

Main clinical manifestations: fever, aversion to wind, perspiration, slow and superficial pulse, dry and itching throat, cough, nasal obstruction and discharge.

These symptoms are due to damage by exogenous pathogenic wind to the body surface and the lung. If exogenous pathogenic wind attacks the skin and muscles, the *wei* (defensive) *qi* is damaged and fails to defend the body surface. So perspiration and aversion to wind occur. When *wei qi* fights against exogenous pathogenic wind, fever arises. When the disease locates in the exterior of the body, it causes sweating, thus the pulse is superficial and slow. When exogenous pathogenic wind attacks the lung, its function will become abnormal in the spreading and descending of *qi* and also brings about a dysfunction of body fluid distribution. The clinical manifestations of dry and itching throat, cough, nasal obstruction and discharge occur.

2. Cold

Pathogenic cold is prevalent in winter and as a *yin* pathogenic factor, it is likely to consume *yang qi*. It also has the characteristics of contracture and stagnation. These are described as follows:

1) Pathogenic cold, as a *yin* pathogenic factor, is liable to

consume the *yang qi* of the body, producing cold syndromes. If the pathogenic cold attacks the body surface leading to a closing of the pores and obstruction of the flow of defensive *yang qi*, it is manifested by the symptom of aversion to cold. If pathogenic cold directly attacks the spleen and stomach it leads to the injury of spleen *yang qi* causing dysfunctions of the whole digestive process. The clinical manifestations are vomiting of clear water, diarrhea, coldness and pain of the epigastric and abdominal regions, pain relieved by warmth and aggravated by cold extremities, etc.

2) Pathogenic cold is characterized by contracture and stagnation. Invasion of pathogenic cold may cause contracture of the blood vessels and tendons, and obstruction of *qi* and blood circulation. This manifests as pain of a cold nature. Pathogenic cold may also cause a common cold with symptoms of sore aching joints and headache. Stagnation of cold in the liver channel leads to hernia of a cold nature, coldness, pain, and swelling of the testis. Pathogenic cold may also cause stomach ache, abdominal pain, etc.

Commonly seen syndromes caused by exogenous pathogenic cold are classified into: cold damaging the skin and muscle and cold damaging the spleen and stomach.

Cold Damaging the Skin and Muscle: fever, aversion to cold, no sweating, tense and superficial pulse, cough, asthma, nasal obstruction, nasal discharge, headache, and aching body.

Fever, aversion to cold, no sweating, tense and superficial pulse are caused by exogenous pathogenic cold that has blocked the spreading of *wei* (defensive) *qi*. The lung is closely related to the skin and hair. If exogenous pathogenic cold blocks the body surface and the *wei qi* can not spread, then lung *qi* fails to disperse and descend, causing nasal obstruction and discharge, cough, and asthma. Exogenous pathogenic cold will also obstruct the channels, resulting in the stagnation of *qi* and blood, which manifests as headache and aching body.

Exogenous Pathogenic Cold Injuring the Spleen and Stomach:

vomiting, diarrhea, borborygmus, and abdominal pain.

This group of symptoms is caused by an over-intake of raw and cold food or the exposure of the abdomen to cold. As exogenous pathogenic cold injures the *yang qi* of the spleen and stomach, then the functions of ascending and descending *qi* by the spleen and stomach become disordered, causing a dysfunction of digestion and absorption with the symptoms of vomiting, diarrhea, abdominal pain, borborygmus, etc.

3. Summer-Heat

Summer-heat is the main pathogenic factor occurring only in the summer. It is a *yang* pathogenic factor. Its characteristics are described as follows:

1) Summer-heat is a *yang* pathogenic factor characterized by sweltering heat. If pathogenic summer-heat attacks the body, the clinical manifestations are *yang*-heat syndromes, such as high fever, burning heat sensation of the skin, irritability, forceful and rapid pulse, etc.

2) Summer-heat consumes *qi* and *yin* (body fluid), and is characterized by upward direction and dispersion. Invasion of pathogenic summer-heat to the head region causes dizziness, vertigo, and excessive sweating due to the abnormal opening of the pores. Excessive sweating exhausts the *qi* and body fluid and manifests as thirst with desire to drink, dryness of the lips and tongue, constipation, yellowish and concentrated urine, etc.

3) Pathogenic summer-heat often combines with damp to cause diseases when the temperature and air humidity are very high. If summer humid-heat attacks the body, the manifestations are fever, heavy sensation of the head or even the whole body, stuffiness and fullness of the chest and epigastric regions, nausea, vomiting, abdominal distension, diarrhea, etc.

Pathogenic factors in summer are summer-heat, sun-stroke and summer humid-heat.

Main clinical manifestations of summer-heat: fever, excessive sweating, irritability, thirst with preference for cold drinks, short-ness of breath, lassitude, general weakness, scanty and yellowish urine, rapid and *xu* (weak) pulse.

Main clinical manifestations of sun stroke: dizziness and vom-iting for mild cases; sudden collapse, unconsciousness, profuse and cold sweating, cold extremities, forceful and *xu* pulse for severe cases.

This group of symptoms are caused by strong sun heat that internally affects the body *qi* activity leading to sudden prostra-tion of *qi* and body fluid.

Main clinical manifestations of summer humid-heat: fever, ir-ritability, stuffy chest, nausea, vomiting, anorexia, lassitude, loose stools, yellowish urine, soft pulse, yellow and sticky tongue coating, etc.

The symptoms resulting from summer humid-heat invasion include the common symptoms of summer-heat, such as fever, irritability, yellowish urine, etc., and the symptoms caused by the obstruction of dampened *qi* circulation, such as stuffy chest, nausea, vomiting and anorexia. Furthermore, there are also the symptoms of internal dampness, such as loose stools, soft pulse, sticky tongue coating, etc.

4. Damp

Damp is the main pathogenic factor causing disease in the late summer since it is the most humid and rainy season. It is a *yin* pathogenic factor with the following characteristics:

1) Pathogenic damp stops the functional activity of *qi* and leads to the injury of spleen *yang*. The spleen functions best in a dry environment and is susceptible to dampness, therefore pathogenic damp is liable to attack spleen *yang*. If spleen *yang* is checked by pathogenic damp, it will cause a dysfunction of transportation and transformation, and obstruct the functional activity of *qi*. The following symptoms will occur: distension and fullness of the epigastric and abdominal regions, anorexia, swee-

tish taste in the mouth, loose stool, cold extremities, etc.

2) Pathogenic damp is a substantial pathogenic factor characterized by heaviness, turbidity, viscosity, stagnation, and sluggishness. Invasion by pathogenic damp also causes the symptoms of heaviness, distension and soreness of the trunk and extremities. The secretions and excretions of the patient have foul and turbid features. The disease duration lingers.

3) Pathogenic damp is characterized by a downward direction. It is a *yin* pathogenic factor which often attacks the lower portion of the body. The *Suwen* says, "When damp attacks the body, it will affect the lower portion first."[46] Clinical manifestations are ulceration and edema of the lower extremities, soreness of muscles, and joint pain of the lower limbs, etc.

Commonly seen syndromes caused by pathogenic damp are exterior damp, and damp *bi*.

Main clinical manifestations of exterior damp: fever, aversion to cold, fever not lowered after sweating, heaviness of the body and head, sore aching of the four limbs, white, thin and slippery tongue coating, soft and slow pulse.

Those symptoms are due to the injury of the body surface by pathogenic damp. When there is obstruction by dampness, it damages the *yang qi* of the body, and blocks the defensive *qi*. So fever and aversion to cold appear. Damp is characterized by heaviness, turbidity, and stickiness. Thus fever is not lowered after sweating. Moreover, other manifestations such as heaviness of the body and head, sore aching of the four limbs, slippery tongue coating, and soft pulse occur.

Damp *bi* is one of the *bi* syndromes due to excessive pathogenic damp, also known as fixed *bi* syndrome.

Manifestations of damp bi: continued soreness at one location, aching and heaviness of the joints, motor impairment, and numbness of the skin.

Bi syndromes indicate the obstruction by wind, cold, or damp in the channels which damages the joints, skin, and muscles. Damp is characterized by heaviness and turbidity, so heaviness is fixed in the joints.

5. Dryness

Dryness is the main pathogenic factor in autumn. Its characteristics are as follows:

1) Pathogenic dryness is apt to consume *yin*, especially body fluids. Clinical manifestations are dryness of the mouth, lips and nose, dryness of the tongue, dry, rough and chapped skin, dry stool, etc.

2) Pathogenic dryness is liable to injure the lung. The lung is considered a tender organ which prefers moisture, cleanliness, and descent. If pathogenic dryness attacks the body from the mouth and nose, the *yin* fluid of the lung is likely to be consumed. It may lead to the dysfunction of dispersion and descent, and manifest as dry cough with scanty sputum, sticky mucus causing difficult expectoration, or bloody sputum, etc.

Commonly seen syndromes caused by pathogenic dryness are cool dryness and warm dryness.

Main clinical manifestations of cool dryness: fever, aversion to cold, headache, no sweating, dryness of the mouth and nose, dry skin, cough with scanty or no sputum, dry white and thin tongue coating.

The symptoms of cool dryness are similar to symptoms caused by exogenous pathogenic cold, but are accompanied with the symptom of body fluid insufficiency.

Main clinical manifestations of warm dryness: fever, mild aversion to wind and cold, headache, scanty perspiration, dry cough, or cough with a small amount of sticky sputum, dry skin, thirst, irritability, red tongue tip and sides, and dry scanty tongue coating. The warm dryness syndrome is similar to the mild heat syndrome, indicating that the body fluid is exhausted.

6. Fire Heat or Mild Heat

Fire, heat, and mild heat are *yang* pathogenic factors. They are of the same nature but differ in intensity. Fire is the outcome of extreme heat. Mild heat is the least severe. These types of heat are sometimes termed pathogenic fire-heat or pathogenic mild heat and are characterized by an upward flaring and damaging of *yin*, with a tendency to disturb the blood system. The following are some special features:

1) Fire is characterized by upward flaring. Clinical manifestations are fever, thirst, profuse sweating, etc. If pathogenic fire travels inward to attack the mind, it causes irritability, anxiety, insomnia, or even mania, unconsciousness, and delirium in severe cases. Since pathogenic fire is likely to flare upward, the clinical manifestations may be mostly on the head and facial regions, such as a swelling and pain of the gums due to extreme stomach fire, ulcers of the tongue and mouth, headache, and redness, pain and swelling of the eyes.

2) Pathogenic fire is liable to consume *yin* fluid. Manifestations are fever, aversion to heat, accompanied by thirst with desire for drinks (especially cold drinks), dryness of throat and mouth, constipation, yellowish urine, etc.

3) Pathogenic fire may disturb the blood and cause extravasation. Mild cases will only have rapid pulse due to acceleration of blood circulation. In severe cases, the blood vessels and collaterals may be damaged, manifesting various hemorrhagic symptoms, such as vomiting of blood (hematemesis), nose bleeds (epistaxis), blood in the urine or stool, excessive menstrual flow, skin eruptions, external boils and ulcers, etc. The common syndrome caused by fire (heat) at the early stage is exterior-heat syndrome.

Main clinical manifestations: fever, mild aversion to cold, headache, sore throat, thirst, yellowish urine, dry stool, red tip and sides of the tongue, superficial and rapid pulse, etc. These symptoms are due to the invasion of fire (heat) on the body surface which consumes body fluids.

This concludes the discussion of the effect of the six exogenous pathological factors on the body. In general, these factors first damage the body surface and then manifest an exterior syndrome with the symptoms of fever and aversion to cold.

Section 2
Pestilential Factors

In addition to the six pathogenic factors, there is another category known as pestilential factors which is the source of epidemic disease. Its nature is similar to pathogenic heat and summer heat, but more pernicious and more fierce in pathogenicity; it is usually accompanied by pathogenic damp. Pestilential diseases are epidemical and dangerous, with rapid drastic changes as seen in smallpox, plague, cholera, and most acute contagious diseases.

Section 3
Seven Emotional Factors

Traditional Chinese medicine emphasizes the relation between diseases and mental activities. Emotional mental activities are categorized as the seven emotional factors: joy, anger, melancholy, worry, grief, fear, and fright. They are the main pathogenic factors of endogenous diseases.

The seven pathogenic emotions are physiological reflections of the human mental state or are induced by various environmental stimulation. Under normal conditions these physiological phenomena will not cause disease. However, if the emotions are too stressful and constant, or the patient is too sensitive to stimulation, then they may induce acute and long-standing changes which result in diseases. Pathogenic emotional factors are considered capable of disturbing the functional activities of *qi*, for example, according to an ancient saying, "Anger makes the *qi* rush upward, overjoy makes the *qi* circulate slowly, grief consumes *qi*, fear causes *qi* to flow downward, fright makes *qi* flow disorderly, overthinking leads to *qi* stagnation."

Different pathogenic emotional factors also selectively damage certain *zang* or *fu* organs. For example, anger injures the liver, overjoy injures the heart, grief and melancholy injure the lung, overthinking injures the spleen, fright and fear injure the kidney. Although emotional pathogenic factors respectively injure the five *zang*, they are mainly related to the heart. The *Lingshu* says, "The heart is the monarch of the five *zang* and six *fu* organs.... Therefore, grief and melancholy also disturb the heart, and a disturbance of the heart leads to the affection of the five *zang* and six *fu* organs."[47] Clinically, the pathological changes of internal organs caused by the seven emotional factors are mostly seen in three of the *zang* organs, namely, the liver, heart, and spleen.

Section 4
Other Pathogenic Factors

Besides the previously mentioned pathogenic factors there are also pathogenic factors relating to irregular food intake, over-strain and stress or insufficient physical exertion, traumatic injuries, parasites, and pathological products such as phlegm-humor and blood stasis.

1. Irregular Diet

Overeating or hunger. Voracious eating or hunger may give rise to disease. Hunger causes malnutrition and leads to an insufficient supply of *qi* and blood, which causes general body weakness. Overeating damages the digestive and absorptive functions, and manifests the symptoms of epigastric and abdominal distension and pain, belching, acid regurgitation, anorexia, vomiting, diarrhea, etc.

Partiality for a particular kind of food: Food intake should be varied. In this way necessary nutrient substances are guaranteed. Partiality to a particular food may bring on disease due to insufficient nutrients. For example: long-term intake of polished white rice may cause beriberi; long-term drinking of iodine-deficient water may cause goiter; indulgence in spicy or boiling hot food may give rise to dryness of the mouth, halitosis, diabetes, etc.; indulgence in smoking, alcoholic drinks, or greasy and highly flavored food may produce pathological phlegm indigestion, stuffy chest, excessive sputum, or boils and ulcers.

Intake of contaminated food: Eating contaminated, poisonous, or stale food (food poisoning) may impair stomach and intestinal functioning causing clinical manifestations such as epigastric and abdominal distension and pain, nausea, vomiting, borborygmus, diarrhea, etc.

Over-strain and stress or deficient physical exertion: Lack of physical exertion may cause retardation of *qi* and blood circulation, unhealthy *zang-fu* organs, general weakness, lassitude, anorexia, dizziness, palpitation, insomnia, etc., also a liability to contract diseases caused by exogenous pathogenic factors. Prolonged over-strain may bring on lassitude, weakness and tiredness of the four extremities, dizziness, hypersomnia, palpitation, spontaneous sweating, asthma or dyspnea due to physical exertion.

In addition, traditional Chinese medicine considers that excessive sexual activity consumes the kidney essence manifested by soreness and weakness of the knees, lumbago, dizziness and vertigo, ringing in the ears, lassitude and listlessness, or even spermatorrhea, impotence, and leukorrhea.

2. Traumatic Injuries and Parasites

Traumatic injuries include incisions, gunshot and sword wounds, scalds and burns, contusions, sprains or animal stings and bites. Mild cases that only sustain injuries to the skin include pain, bleeding, bruises, and hematoma due to the obstruction of blood vessels. While severe cases may include injuries to the tendons, bones, and internal organs manifesting as joint dislocation, fracture, hemorrhage due to rupture of the internal organs, prostration, etc.

3. Phlegm-Humor and Blood Stagnation

Phlegm-Humor: Phlegm-humor can form due to the accumulation of body fluids, therefore it has a close relationship to functional disorders of the lung, spleen, and kidney which control water metabolism. It may also be produced by an over-indulgence in alcohol or fatty and highly flavored foods, leading to stagnation of liver *qi* and derangement of the functional activities of *qi*.

Blood Stagnation: Under normal conditions, blood circulates continually within the blood vessels at a certain speed. Any retarded circulation of blood or extravasated blood in spaces between the tissues may form blood stasis. Its syndromes are characterized as follows:

Pain: The pain location is fixed with local tenderness and has a stabbing or boring sensation.

Hemorrhage: Blood stagnation prevents normal flow inside the vessels causing extravasation and hemorrhage. The blood is often deep red or dark purplish.

Ecchymosis or Petechia: Blood stagnation subcutaneously forms ecchymosis or petechiae accompanied by local pain. Initially they present a red color, then change to purple or yellow, finally disappearing. If the tongue proper is purple, or ecchymosis or petechiae are present, this is significant in the diagnosis of diseases caused by blood stagnation.

Mass Tumor: Most mass tumors, especially large lumps in the abdominal cavity, are considered to be related to stagnation of the blood. The location of the tumors should be fixed and unmovable, accompanied by pain.

Chapter 6
Methods of Diagnosis

The human body is an organic entity, so local pathological changes may affect the whole body. Moreover, the pathological changes of the internal organs may reflect on the body surface.

Diagnostic methods in traditional Chinese medicine include four basic methods: inspection, auscultation and olfaction, inquiry and palpation. The case history, symptoms, and signs gained through those four diagnostic methods are analyzed and generalized to find the causes, nature, and interrelations of the disease, and to provide evidence for the further differentiation of syndromes. The four diagnostic methods are therefore indispensable and important steps in the differentiation and treatment of syndromes.

Section 1
Inspection

Inspection is a method to examine the patient by observation of the expression, appearance, color, and abnormal changes of secretion and excretion, etc.

1. Observation of the Mind

This is to observe the patient's spirit, clearness of consciousness, coordination and vigour of movements, and keenness of response in order to judge the excess or deficiency of *yin, yang, qi,* and blood in the *zang-fu* organs and make a prognosis of the disease condition.

Strength of Spirit: The patient is in good spirits, the body resistance and functions of the *zang-fu* organs are normal, therefore the patient has a good prognosis. Generally speaking, the patient is in good spirits, behaves normally with a sparkle in the eye, and has a keen response.

Loss of Spirit: The patient is spiritless, indifferent in expression, has dull eyes and a sluggish response, or may even be unconscious or have a mental disturbance. This shows damage to the body resistance, a severe disease condition, and a poor prognosis.

2. Observation of the Complexion

Observe the color and luster of the facial region. Generally, a lustrous complexion with normal color indicates ample *qi* and blood, and a mild disease with a good prognosis. If the complexion is deep in color and withered, this indicates a serious disease condition with damage to the *qi* and essence, and a difficult treatment with poor prognosis.

White Color: A white color is the sign of a *qi* and blood deficiency. A pale complexion indicates a *yin* excess with *yang* deficiency. A *qi* deficiency manifests a lusterless and pale complexion and is accompanied by swelling. A pale emaciated face indicates a blood deficiency. A sudden pale complexion with cold sweat is the sign of sudden prostration of *yang qi* due to febrile diseases caused by exogenous pathogenic wind-cold.

Yellowish Color. A yellowish color is the sign of spleen deficiency and damp accumulation. A complexion that is yellowish, withered and lusterless indicates a *qi* deficiency of the spleen and stomach. A yellowish, flabby complexion is the sign of damp accumulation due to spleen dysfunction of transportation and transformation. The yellow color of the face, eyes, and skin indicates jaundice. In traditional Chinese medicine a bright orange yellow is diagnosed as *yang* jaundice caused by pathogenic damp-heat; dark yellow is *yin* jaundice due to pathogenic cold-damp.

Red Color. Redness indicates excessively full blood vessels due to excessive heat. A red complexion is mostly due to the fever of a common cold, or may be a heat syndrome due to excessive *yang* in the *zang-fu* organs. Malar flush with bright red color indicates *xu* heat syndromes due to *yin* deficiency and *yang* preponderance.

Bluish Color. Bluish color indicates syndromes of cold, pain, and blood stasis or convulsion, and is the manifestation of *qi* and blood obstruction in the channels. Pathogenic cold causes stagnation of *qi* and blood leading to pain. Children's high fever also shows a bluish complexion, the symptom of acute convulsion.

Black Color. Black color indicates kidney deficiency, humor accumulation, and blood stasis. This is the manifestation of excessive cold and water, or stagnation of *qi* and blood. If the complexion is as black as bronze, it is mostly due to an extreme weakness of kidney *yang* and cold accumulation manifesting as *xu*-cold syndromes. A dark gray color around the eyes denotes phlegm-humor syndrome due to kidney deficiency. This leads to a dysfunction of the water metabolism or leukorrhea, due to the downward flowing of kidney essence. A dark gray malar can be seen in patients with frequent urination due to kidney deficiency. A dark gray complexion indicates prolonged stagnation of blood such as a consumptive disease with blood deficiency accompanied by menoplania or amenia.

3. Observation of the Tongue

Tongue Proper
Pale Tongue: Indicates *xu* and cold syndromes or symptoms due to *yang qi* deficiency and insufficiency of *qi* and blood.

Red Tongue: Indicates heat syndromes, mostly *shi* types of disease caused by interior heat, or symptoms of fire preponderance due to *yin* deficiency.

Deep Red Tongue: Denotes the excessive heat seen in febrile disease due to invasion of exogenous pathogenic heat which has been transmitted from the exterior to the interior of the body. It also can be seen in miscellaneous diseases due to a preponderance of fire caused by *yin* deficiency, or seen in diseases of accumulated fire in the liver channel.

Purplish Tongue: Shows the syndrome of blood stagnation. A tongue with purplish spots or petechiae also indicates blood stagnation.

Tongue Appearance
Flabby Tongue: A flabby tongue body with teeth marks on the margin and pale in color indicates a *yang* deficiency of the spleen and kidney leading to accumulation and obstruction of phlegm-dampness. A flabby tongue with a deep red color indicates excessive pathogenic heat attacking the heart and spleen.

Thin and Small Tongue: This indicates consumption and deficiency of blood and *yin*. A thin and small tongue with a pale color denotes deficiency of both *qi* and blood. A thin dry tongue with a deep red color is mainly due to a preponderance of fire and great exhaustion of body fluids.

Rigid Tongue: Seen in febrile diseases due to the invasion of exogenous pathogenic heat transmitted into the pericardium or due to an obstruction of pathogenic phlegm. It may also be seen in high fever leading to consumption of body fluids and preponderance of pathogenic heat. It is a prodrome of wind-stroke (cerebral stroke).

Deviated Tongue: This is a prodrome of wind-stroke.

Cracked Tongue: Cracks on the tongue with deep red color indicate excessive heat. A cracked pale tongue indicates insufficiency of *yin* and blood. However, a cracked tongue of long term duration without any other symptoms can be considered normal.

Tongue Coating

In the first place, the properties of tongue coating should be examined.

Thinness and Thickness: Generally, if substantial pathogenic factors such as damp, phlegm or food accumulation occur and cause obstruction, they further affect the spleen and stomach leading to the ascent of turbid *qi* and forming of a thick tongue coating. A white thin tongue coating is formed if nonsubstantial pathogenic factors such as wind, heat, dryness, or cold attack the body; or if the pathogenic factors stay on the body surface; or if body resistance is weak during the disease development.

Moistness and Dryness: The normal tongue coating is moist, which indicates that plenty of body fluid is flowing upward. If the tongue coating is dry, it is due to body fluids failing to moisten the tongue. A dry tongue coating may also be present in some febrile diseases where pathogenic heat consumes the body fluid. A slippery tongue coating may be due to pathogenic damp-humor floating over the tongue surface.

Sticky and Curdled Tongue Coating: A sticky coating is due to hyperactivity of endogenous pathogenic phlegm and damp rising tot he tongue, and is mostly seen in diseases caused by pathogenic damp-heat or phlegm-humor. A curdled tongue coating is the outcome of food accumulation in the stomach

110

leading to the ascent of turbid *qi* to the tongue surface. It is also seen in disease caused by phlegm-damp.

Peeled Tongue Coating: Mostly due to deficiency of *qi* and *yin*. If peeled tongue is accompanied by a sticky coating, it indicates a complicated disease condition to which the body resistance is weakened.

No Tongue Coating: Changes in the tongue coating indicate fluctuation in the disease condition. For example, if a *qi* deficiency of the stomach is manifested by no tongue coating at an early stage, the tongue coating will reappear after the stomach *qi* is recovered. If a disease has no tongue coating, then suddenly appears, this indicates a perversive flow of stomach *qi*, or excessive pathogenic heat. If a disease has a tongue coating at the beginning which disappears abruptly, this indicates stomach *yin* fluid has decreased. If a thick coating gradually turns into a thin white coating, this indicates that pathogenic *qi* is being gradually weakened, and the disease condition is becoming milder.

Generally, an observation of the thinness and thickness of the tongue coating will indicate the depth of pathogenic *qi*. The tongue's moistness or dryness shows the body fluid condition. The degree of curdling and stickiness of the tongue coating indicates the dampness of the stomach and spleen. The appearance or disappearance of tongue coating signifies the cure or worsening of the disease condition.

Color of Tongue Coating

White Coating: Indicates exterior-cold syndromes. A white and thin coating is seen mostly in exterior syndromes, while a white and thick coating appears in interior-cold syndromes. If there is a powder-like whitish coating covering the tongue surface, it is caused by the internal accumulation of summer-humid heat and is usually seen at the onset of pestilential diseases.

Yellow Coating: Indicates interior and heat syndromes. A light yellow tongue coating is seen in cases of slight fever. A deep yellow color indicates high fever. Brownish tongue coatings represent an accumulation of pathogenic heat.

Grayish Coating: Denotes interior-heat syndrome or interior-cold syndrome. A grayish black and slippery coating on the tongue usually indicates a symptom-complex due to cold-damp in the interior. A grayish, yellow, and sticky tongue coating usually indicates the accumulation of damp-heat. Grayish and dry tongue coatings are usually due to the consumption of body fluid by excessive heat.

Black Coating: This is often seen at the serious and dangerous stage of disease, and indicates extreme heat or cold. A black, yellow, and dry coating with thorns on the tongue surface usually denotes consumption of body fluid by extreme heat. A black and slippery tongue coating shows excessive cold due to *yang* deficiency.

Section 2
Auscultation and Olfaction

Auscultation (listening) and olfaction (smelling) are two methods used to diagnose a disease.

1. Listening

Listening to the Voice
Speaking Voice: Generally, speaking in a loud and sonorous voice indicates syndromes of heat or *shi* type, while a feeble, low voice indicates syndromes of the cold or *xu* type.

Disordered Speaking: Speaking incoherently and loudly or deliriously indicates *shi* syndrome. Speaking verbosely, feebly, and intermittently indicates syndromes of the *xu* type. Muttering to oneself denotes *qi* deficiency of the heart. Stuttering speech suggests upward disturbance of wind-phlegm.

Listening to the Respiration

Feeble Breathing: Feeble breathing accompanied by shortness of breath usually indicates *xu* syndromes.

Coarse Breathing: Forceful breathing with a coarse voice belongs to the *shi* heat type syndromes. Asthma with feeble, short breathing is a category of *xu* type asthma.

Listening to the Cough

Coarse coughing usually indicates *shi* type syndromes. A low cough with weak breathing indicates *xu* syndromes.

2. Smelling

Foul breath is due to pathogenic heat in the stomach, indigestion, caries, and an unclean mouth. Sour breath indicates food accumulation in the stomach.

The offensive smell of a secretion or excretion including stool, urine, sputum, pus, leukorrhea, etc., usually indicates heat syndromes of the *shi* type. A stinking smell usually indicates cold syndromes of the *xu* type.

3. Inquiring

Inquiring involves asking the patient or the patient's companion about the disease condition to assist diagnosis.

Because the chief complaint of the patient is of primary importance, the main information dealing with the problem must be carefully solicited. It is necessary to grasp the important clinical data as well as to get a general understanding of the patient's disease condition. The main catagories of concern are:

Chills and Fever

Aversion to Cold and Fever: At the beginning of a disease, aversion to cold and Fever occurs simultaneously. This indicates exterior syndromes due to invasion by exogenous pathogenic factors.

The exterior syndromes due to invasion by exogenous pathogenic cold and wind are characterized by severe aversion to cold, mild fever accompanied by an absence of thirst, no sweat, headache, general pain, superficial and tense pulse, etc.

The exterior syndromes due to invasion by exogenous pathogenic wind-heat are characterized by severe fever, mild aversion to cold accompanied by thirst, sweating, sore throat, superficial and rapid pulse, etc.

Alternating Chills and Fever. This particular symptom occurs when exogenous pathogenic factors are in between the exterior and interior of the body, accompanied by a bitter taste in the mouth, dry throat, fullness of the chest, hypochondrium, etc. If a high fever follows the first occurrence of chills and is complicated with a severe headache which subsides after the fever is gone, this indicates malaria.

Fever Occurring Without Chills

High fever. This is usually due to the transmission of exogenous pathogenic cold from the exterior to the interior, which then changes into heat; or the transmission of exogenous pathogenic heat from exterior to interior resulting in a *shi* type interior-heat syndrome accompanied by profuse sweating, thirst, forceful pulse, etc.

Tidal fever. This is one of the main characteristics of *yin* deficiency or *shi* heat syndrome of the Yangming channel. Tidal fever due to *yin* deficiency often occurs at noon or night, accompanied by a dry red tongue. Tidal fever usually appears at dusk associated with constipation, abdominal distension, penis pain, etc.

Perspiration

Sweat is transformed from evaporated body fluid by the function of *yang qi*. So perspiration has a certain clinical significance in reflecting the status of *yang qi* and body fluid. One should first ask whether the patient has sweat or not. If the patient is sweating, further questioning should be concerned with the characteristics and accompanied symptoms of perspiration.

Sweating of No Sweating: Exterior syndromes without sweating are caused by exogenous pathogenic factors. Exterior syndromes with sweating are mostly exterior heat syndromes due to the invasion by exogenous pathogenic wind heat; or they may be exterior *xu* syndromes due to exogenous pathogenic wind.

Night Sweating: Is usually the manifestation of *yin* deficiency, accompanied by tidal fever, flushed malar, red tongue proper with scanty coating, thready and rapid pulse.

Spontaneous Sweating: This is a sign of *qi* or *yang* deficiency associated with fear of cold, lassitude, etc.

Profuse Sweating: Excessive sweating together with high fever, thirst with desire for cold drinks, forceful pulse, etc. belongs to interior *shi* heat syndrome. This is the outcome of excessive *yang* and heat compelling the outward flow of sweat. Dripping with sweat accompanied by lassitude, feckless breathing, cold extremities, and feeble pulse indicates the total prolapse of *yang qi*, also known as "sweating from exhaustion."

Sweating of the Head: Caused by heat in the upper *jiao* or damp heat in the middle *jiao*. If it is caused by the heat in the upper *jiao*, it will be accompanied by irritability, thirst, yellow tongue coating, superficial and rapid pulse. If it is the result of damp heat accumulation, it will be associated with heaviness and tiredness of the body, dysuria, yellowish and sticky tongue coating, etc.

Food and Drink, Appetite, and Taste

No Appetite: This is a symptom caused by the dysfunction of transformation and transportation of the spleen. Symptoms are emaciation due to chronic disease, poor appetite, loose stool, lassitude, and pale tongue proper with a thin white coating. If anorexia is associated with fullness of the chest, abdominal distension, thick and sticky tongue coating, then it is caused by the obstruction of pathogenic damp in the spleen.

Food Repulsion: This is usually due to the accumulation of food in the stomach and intestines. It is often accompanied by distension and fullness of the epigastrium and abdomen, acid regurgitation, and a thick and sticky tongue coating.

Quick Hunger: This is due to strong stomach fire and causes fast digestion.

Hunger and Anorexia Combined: This is due to injury of stomach *yin* and disturbance of *xu* heat.

Craving for Dirt Due to Intestinal Parasites: This is common in children, and is a sign of parasitosis accompanied by emaciation, abdominal distension and pain, etc.

Thirst: Whether the patient is thirsty or not often reflects the condition of body fluids. During the process of disease development, if there is no thirst, then the body fluid has not yet been damaged and it indicates a cold syndrome. If the patient is thirsty, it indicates a consumption or stagnation of the body fluid failing to nourish the upper body.

Generally, thirst with a desire for excessive drinking is commonly seen in heat syndromes. Severe thirst with a preference for hot drinks indicates a phlegm-humor obstruction which prevents the upward flow of body fluids. The upward flow of water usually causes vomiting after drinking due to thirst. If the patient is thirsty, but doesn't want to drink, this indicates acute febrile diseases where the pathogenic factors have invaded the nutrient (*ying*) and blood (*xue*) systems of the body. If excessive drinking does not relieve the symptom of thirst and then excessive urination follows, this suggests diabetes.

Taste: Clinically, a bitter taste in the mouth is caused by pathogenic heat, especially the overflowing of heat from the liver and gall bladder. A sweet taste in the mouth is usually due to damp heat in the spleen and stomach. A sour taste is due to the accumulation of heat in the liver and stomach. A sour taste similar to spoiled food indicates injury by the accumulation of food. Tastelessness in the mouth is usually due to the dysfunction of transportation and transformation.

Defecation and Urination

Shape of the Stool: Dry stools shaped like sheep-dung are due to stagnation of heat or exhaustion of body fluid. A mucous stool is a sign of excessive damp caused by spleen deficiency. Loose bowels following dry stool are due to a dysfunction of the spleen and stomach, and an imbalance between dryness and dampness. Stools which are sometimes dry and sometimes loose are usually due to liver *qi* stagnation and spleen deficiency. Liquid stools with undigested food are due to the *yang* deficiency of the spleen and kidney. Diarrhea with yellow watery stool and burning of the anus is caused by damp heat in the stomach and intestines. Formed stools with undigested food and foul smell are the result of food accumulation.

The Color of the Stool: Tarry stools are the symptoms of hemorrhaging in the spleen and stomach. Bloody and pussy stools are a sign of dysentery.

The Smell of the Stool: Sour stinking stools are due to the accumulation of heat. A rotten egg stink is due to food accumulation.

The Sensation of Defecation: A burning sensation in the anus during defecation is due to pathogenic heat in the rectum. Mild prolapse of the anus during bowel movements is the outcome of chronic diarrhea due to the sinking of *qi* and spleen deficiency. Tenesmus is a sign of dysentery due to *qi* stagnation in the intestines. Fragmentary defection is a manifestation of the liver failing to cause a free condition for *qi*. Diarrhea occurring soon after abdominal pain, and pain relieved after bowel movements, are signs of food accumulation. Pain not relieved after bowel movements is a sign of spleen deficiency and liver preponderance resulting in "liver-wood subjugating the spleen-earth."

The Color of Urine: Deep yellow urine indicates heat, while clear and profuse urine indicates cold. Turbid urine or a mixture of urine with sperm denotes the downward flowing of damp heat. Brownish urine indicates that pathogenic heat has injured the blood vessels.

The Amount of Urine: An increased amount of urine indicates kidney *qi* deficiency. A decreased volume of urine is caused by the consumption of body fluid or by dysfunction of *qi* activities causing failure to transform body fluids into urine. Dribbling of urine or retention of urine indicates the exhaustion of kidney *qi* or the downward flowing of damp heat.

The Sensation of Urination: A stabbing pain during urination, accompanied by an urgent and burning feeling, is caused by damp heat. Pain after urination mostly indicates the declining of kidney *qi*. Dribbling urination is due to the non-consolidation of kidney *qi*. Nocturnal enuresis is caused by the deficiency of kidney *qi*. Unconsciousness accompanied by incontinence of urine indicates that the heart has failed to control the mind and the urinary bladder has lost its restrictive capacity.

Pain

Headache: Occipital headache, referring to the nape and the upper back, is a disease of the Taiyang channel. Frontal headache, referring to the supraorbital ridge, indicates a disease of the Yangming channel. Headaches of the temporal region are diseases of the Shaoyang channel. Vertex headache is a pain of the Jueyin channel. Headache related to the teeth is a pain of the Shaoyin channel due to invasion by cold.

Pain of the Chest: This is mostly due to the obstruction of phlegm or blood stasis, leading to *qi* stagnation.

Pain in the Hypochondriac Region: Is caused by obstruction in the liver and gall bladder channel, or by malnutrition of these channels.

Epigastric Pain: Is caused by disorders of the stomach.

Abdominal Pain: Lower lateral abdominal pain is caused by *qi* stagnation of the liver, obstruction of the liver channel, or appendicitis or hernia. Pain around the umbilicus is seen in parasitosis, food accumulation, constipation, etc. Lower abdominal pain and distension is caused by dysuria and/or retention of urine. If there are no complicated urination symptoms, the usual cause is retention of blood in the lower *jiao*.

Low Back Pain: Is mostly due to a deficiency of the kidney, invasion by cold damp, or blood stagnation in the channels.

Pain of the Limbs: Pain may appear in joints, muscles, or channels and collaterals due to the invasion of exogenous pathogenic factors.

The Nature of Pain: A wandering pain associated with numbness or itching is due to invasion by pathogenic wind. Pain associated with heaviness and soreness is most often caused by pathogenic damp. Severe pain with a cold feeling or fear of cold is caused by pathogenic cold. Pain accompanied by redness, swelling, and heat or fear of heat is due to pathogenic fire (heat). Distending pain or referred pain is caused by *qi* stagnation. Pain which is aggravated by pressure relates to the *shi* type of symptom complex. Pain which is alleviated by pressure is related to the *xu* type of symptom complex.

Sleep

Insomnia associated with palpitation, dreams and nervousness is usually caused by the insufficiency of blood nourishing the heart. Insomnia accompanied by restlessness in the mind and difficulty in falling asleep indicates *yin* deficiency leading to preponderance of fire. Insomnia complicated by bitter taste, vomiting saliva, palpitation, irritability, and an inability to fall asleep indicates the internal disturbance of phlegm-fire. Insomnia due to the disharmony of the stomach indicates a derangement of stomach *qi* leading to restlessness in the mind during sleep.

Hypersomnia is commonly seen in febrile diseases caused by exogenous pathogenic factors; in *qi* deficiency caused by chronic diseases; in failure of the spleen *yang* to ascend due to the obstruction of damp; or in the condition of *yang* deficiency leading to excessive *yin*.

Menses and Leukorrhea

Antedated Menstruation: Red color and an excessive amount

indicates heat syndrome. Light color, post-menstrual pain in the lower abdomen is most often due to a deficiency of both *qi* and blood.

Postdated Menstruation: Dark purple menstrual flow with clots, and premenstrual abdominal pain, most often indicates cold syndromes or blood stasis. Postdated menstruation with a scanty light-coloured flow indicates blood deficiency.

Indefinite Menstruation: If it is associated with dysmenorrhea or distension of the breasts before menstruation, it is caused by the stagnation of liver *qi*.

Amenorrhea: Many factors may cause amenorrhea, such as pregnancy, blood stasis, blood exhaustion, consumptive diseases, *qi* stagnation in the liver, etc.

Incessant Menstrual Flow: If it is dark purple color with clots and abdominal pain, this indicates deficiency of the *chong* and *ren* channels, or failure of blood control by the spleen due to sinking *qi* of the middle *jiao*.

Leukorrhea: Thin and whitish leukorrhea with little odor indicates deficiency of the spleen and kidney. Excessive yellowish and thick leukorrhea with offensive smell indicates the downward flow of damp heat.

4. Palpation

Palpation is a method of diagnosis using the hand to touch, feel, and press certain areas of the body to ascertain the patient's disease condition. Generally there are two types: pulse feeling and body palpation.

Pulse Feeling

In traditional Chinese medicine the pulse is considered as having three divisions: *cun*, *guan*, and *chi*. A normal pulse is neither superficial nor deep, neither quick nor slow, and it beats in medium frequency, i.e., 4-5 beats per breath, with a regular rhythm.

Methods of Diagnosis

To feel the pulse correctly, place the patients hand comfortably on a cushion with the palm facing upward. First, the practitioner should put their middle finger on the *guan* division, then the index and ring fingers should naturally fall on the *cun* and *chi* divisions. Finger force should at first be light, then moderate and finally heavy to get a general picture of the depth, rhythm, strength, and form of the pulse. An even force should be applied on the three regions. Through comparisons of the three regions, the practitioner can gain a correct impression of the pulse as a whole. A normal pulse is of moderate frequency, i.e., 4-5 beats per breath, regular rhythm, even and forceful.

The following are abnormal pulses commonly seen in the clinic:

Floating Pulse (fumai): When the pulse is pressed lightly it appears under the finger, and when pressed heavily it becomes weak. It often occurs in the early stages of diseases caused by exogenous pathogenic wind cold and heat, i.e., exterior syndromes. If it is seen in patients who are suffering from prolonged chronic diseases, it indicates a dangerous site where the *yang qi* of the body flows outward.

Deep Pulse (chimai): No clear pulse is felt by superficial pressure, only by heavy pressure. This indicates an interior syndrome.

Rapid Pulse (sumai): The pulse beats rapidly at a rate higher than the normal 5 beats per breath (i.e., more than 90 times per minute). This indicates a heat syndrome.

Xu Type Pulse (xumai): If the pulses of the three regions are weak and forceless, this indicates *xu* type syndromes. These are mostly caused by both *qi* and blood deficiencies and are seen during the process of chronic diseases.

Shi Type Pulse (shimai): If the pulses of the three regions are forceful with both light and heavy pressure, *shi* type syndromes are present.

Slippery pulse (huamai): If the pulse is smooth and flowing, like a pearl rolling on a plate, this indicates excessive phlegm, retention of food, or *shi* heat type syndromes.

Rough Pulse (semai): This pulse is uneven and has a roughness similar to scraping bamboo with a knife. It indicates a deficiency of blood and essence, *qi* stagnation, and blood stasis.

Fine Pulse (ximai): This pulse is as fine as a silk thread, and indicates exhaustion of *qi* and blood.

Full Pulse (hongmai): This pulse beats like a dashing wave, with one rising wave following another. It indicates excessive heat.

Wiry Pulse (xuanmai): This pulse is straight and long, like a tremulous music string, seen usually in diseases of liver, gall bladder, pain, or phlegm-humor.

Tense Pulse (jinmai): The pulse is taut and forceful, like a tightly stretched cord, and occurs in diseases caused by cold, pain, or retention of food.

Hollow Pulse (koumai): This pulse is floating, large, and empty inside, feeling like a scallion stalk. It indicates a massive loss of blood and essence.

Hesitant Pulse (cumai): This pulse is rapid with irregular intermittent beats. It indicates excessive *yang* and *shi* heat, *qi* stagnation, pathogenic phlegm mixture with cold, blood stasis, etc.

Knotted Pulse (jiemai): This pulse is slow and uneven with irregular intervals. It indicates excessive *yin*, *qi* stagnation, pathogenic phlegm mixture with cold, blood stasis, etc.

Intermittent Pulse (daimai): This pulse is slow with regular intervals. It indicates *qi* exhaustion of the *zang* organs, or syndromes of wind and pain caused by emotional pathogenic fright and fear.

Body Palpation

This is a diagnostic method to ascertain abnormal changes in the body and to determine the location and nature of the disease through palpation and finger pressure.

Palpating the Skin and Muscle: Generally, if there is excessive pathogenic heat in the body, the patient will usually have heat on the body surface. *Yang qi* deficiency has a cold body surface on palpation. If the surface feels hot on first palpation becoming slightly hotter when you palpate longer, this indicates that the pathogenic heat has proceeded from the exterior to the interior of the body. Body palpation showing moist and smooth skin demonstrates that the body fluid is not yet damaged. If the skin and nails are very dry, this indicates consumption of the body fluids. If body palpation shows swelling and further pressure makes a depression, this indicates edema. If a depression appears on pressure and disappears after taking the hand away, this indicates *qi* distension. Palpating the skin can also indicate the patient's sweat condition.

Palpating Hands and Feet: Coldness of the four extremities is mostly due to *yang* deficiency and excessive pathogenic cold. An overheating of the four extremities indicates excessive heat. Coldness of the four extremities with heat in the chest and abdomen is due to the retention of internal heat preventing the flow of *yang qi* outward. Heat in the dorsum of the hand is a sign of disease caused by exogenous pathogenic factors.

Palpating the Epigastrium and Abdomen: If the patient has fullness and distension of the hypochondrium, palpation may demonstrate hardness and pain in this region. This is known as an accumulation of excessive pathogenic factors in the chest of the *xu* type. If the hardness extends over a large area in the chest, it is due to phlegm-humor.

Palpation of the abdomen showing abdominal distention with a tympanitic note on percussion, but with normal urination, indicates *qi* tympanites. Abdominal distension with a splashing sound like water, and accompanying dysuria indicates water tympanites or ascites. If hand pressure relieves the abdominal pain, it is considered to be a *xu* type; if the pain is made worse by pressure, it is a *shi* type. Immovable hard masses in the abdomen with pain fixed in a certain area are due to blood stasis. However, if the patient feels that lumps sometimes appear and disappear with unfixed pain, and palpation of the abdomen shows they do not exist, then this is due to *qi* stagnation.

Palpating Channels and Points: Clinical practice proves that in some diseases there may occur tenderness or abnormal reactions along the courses of the affected channels or at certain points. These signs have significance in diagnosis by palpation, especially in acupuncture treatment. For example, there may be tenderness at Pt. Zhongfu (Lu. 1) or Pt. Shufu (K. 27), which are closely related to the disorders of the lung and trachea. In diseases of the heart and stomach, tenderness may occur at Pt. Jugue (Ren 14), Pt. Zhongwan (Ren 12), Pt. Burong (St. 19), or Pt. Liangmen (St. 21). In disorders of the liver and gall bladder, tenderness may be at Pt. Qimen (Liv. 14) and Pt. Riyue (G.B. 24). In diseases of the spleen, tenderness may occur at Pt. Zhangmen (Liv. 13) and Pt. Huangmen (U.B. 51). In disorders of the kidney, Pt. Jingmen (G.B. 25) and Pt. Zhishi (U.B. 52) may have tenderness. Tenderness at Pt. Tianshu (St. 25). Pt. Daju (St. 27) and Pt. Fujie (Sp. 14) may be closely related to disorders of the intestines. Tenderness at Pt. Guanyuan (Ren 4), Pt. Qihai (Ren 6) and Pt. Zhongji (Ren 3) may have a close relation with disorders of the urinogenital system. When there are abnormal reactions appearing at the above points, they may reflect pathological changes of the related *zang* or *fu* organs.

Chapter 7
Differentiation of
Syndromes

Differentiation of syndromes is a method of understanding and diagnosing disease by the theories of traditional Chinese medicine. The diagnostic procedure involves an analysis of the clinical data regarding symptoms, physical signs, and disease history, together with information obtained from an application of the four diagnostic methods. Only correct differentiation can give a correct diagnosis and thus a suitable method of treatment. Therefore the four diagnostic methods are the basis of the differentiation of syndromes, and the differentiation of syndromes is the basis of clinical treatment. Furthermore, the effect of clinical treatment is the criteria of judgment for the correctness of the deduced differentiation. These three aspects form an organic connection — a basic law of diagnosis and treatment in traditional Chinese medicine, that is, "applying the treatment on the basis of differentiating syndromes."

There are a variety of methods for differentiating syndromes: differentiation according to the eight principles; according to the theory of *zang-fu* organs; according to the theory of six channels; according to the theory of *wei, qi, ying*, and *xue*; according to the theory of the *sanjiao*; according to the theory of *qi*, blood, and body fluids; according to etiology, etc. Each of these methods has its own characteristics and emphasis, while in clinical practice they are interrelated with each other and complement each other. Regarding content, the differentiation of syndromes according to the eight principles is the dominant procedure and the differentiation of syndromes according to the theory of *zang-fu* organs is the basis of all the other methods. Other methods of differentiation can be separated from these two. Therefore this book mainly introduces the method of differentiating syndromes according to the eight principles and the theory of *zang-fu* organs. The method of differentiating syndromes according to the theory of channels and collaterals has discussed in Chapter IV.

Section 1
Differentiation of Syndromes According to the Eight Principles

The eight principles of differentiating syndromes are *yin* and *yang*, exterior (*biao*) and interior (*li*), *xu* (deficiency) and *shi* (excess), and cold and heat. These eight basic syndromes signify the location of pathological changes, the nature of disease, the condition of body resistance and pathogenic factors. These are the general principles for differentiation of syndromes and no matter how complex the disease, the eight principles can be used to give an analysis and differentiation.

1. Exterior and Interior

Exterior and interior are two principles indicating the depth and development of disease. Exterior syndromes refer to the pathological changes and syndromes which are caused by the invasion of the body surface by exogenous pathogenic factors.

Exterior syndromes are usually acute occurrences, superficially located, and with a short duration. The main clinical manifestations are aversion to cold and fever, thin and white tongue coating, floating pulse, etc.

Interior syndromes result from the transmission of exogenous pathogenic factors into the interior or from the dysfunction of the *zang-fu* organs.

Interior syndromes have extensive indications. Regarding the occurrence of disease, there are three conditions:

a. Interior syndromes may occur due to transmission of exogenous pathogenic factors into the interior after lengthy contact.

b. They may result from direct attack on the *zang-fu* organs by exogenous pathogenic factors.

c. Dysfunction of *zang-fu* organs may also be due to interior syndromes.

2. Cold and Heat

Cold and heat are two principles for differentiating the nature of disease.

Cold syndromes are pathological changes and symptoms caused by exogenous pathogenic cold or constitutional *yang* deficiency. Clinical manifestations of cold syndromes are: aversion to cold and preference for warmth; tastelessness in the mouth; absence of thirst; pallor; cold extremities; clear and profuse urine; loose stool; pale tongue proper with a white slippery coating; slow pulse, etc. These are all signs of excessive *yin*.

Heat syndromes are caused by exogenous pathogenic heat or constitutional *yin* deficiency. The symptoms of heat syndromes include: fever; preference for cold; thirst with preference for cold drinks; flushed cheeks and redness of the eyes; yellowish and scanty urine; constipation; red tongue proper with a dry yellowish coating; rapid pulse, etc. These are signs of preponderant *yang*.

3. *Xu* (deficiency) and *Shi* (Excess)

Xu (deficiency) and *shi* (excess) are two principles which are used to analyze the strength or weakness of body resistance and the pathogenic factors during the process of disease development.

Generally, syndromes of the *xu* type indicate diseases and symptoms caused by the weakness and insufficiency of body resistance. Syndromes of the *shi* type refer to diseases and symptoms induced by an overabundance of exogenous pathogenic factors. *Xu* syndromes are mainly due to an insufficiency of antipathogenic factors when exogenous pathogenic factors are also in a weakened state. *Shi* syndromes are mainly due to an excess of exogenous pathogenic factors, with body resistance not yet weakened. Mixture syndromes of *xu* and *shi* also occur.

Xu syndromes can be further classified into *qi* deficiency, blood deficiency, *yang* deficiency, and *yin* deficiency with varied clinical manifestations. *Shi* syndromes may be caused by *qi* stagnation, blood stasis, phlegm obstruction, stagnancy of water, and parasites with complex clinical manifestations. Different types of *xu* and *shi* syndromes have been introduced in related chapters. The general *xu* syndromes include lassitude, emaciation, sluggishness, pale complexion, palpitation, shortness of breath, spontaneous sweating, night sweating, insomnia, poor memory, loose stool, frequent urination or incontinence of urine, pale tongue proper without coating, thready and weak pulse, etc.

Shi syndromes generally include coarse breathing, irritability, sonorous voice, pain and distension in the chest and abdomen, pain and distension aggravated by pressure, constipation, dysuria, thick and sticky tongue coating, forceful *shi* pulse, etc. However, the patient's body can still remain strong and vigorous.

4. *Yin* and *Yang*

Yin and *yang* are two general principles used to categorize the other six principles, i.e., exterior, heat and *shi* belong to the category of *yang*, while interior, cold, and *xu* belong to *yin*. *Yang* syndromes and *yin* syndromes can be detailed as the collapse of *yin*, collapse of *yang*, *yin xu* (*yin* deficiency), *yang xu* (*yang* deficiency), etc.

Yin xu and yang xu syndromes: *Yin xu* indicates consumption or loss of *yin* fluid. *Yang xu* manifests as the insufficiency of *yang qi*. *Yin xu* syndromes are afternoon fever, malar flush, feverish sensation in the palms and soles, irritability, insomnia, night sweating, dry mouth and throat, scanty and yellowish urine, dry stool, red tongue proper with little coating, and thready and rapid pulse. Since *yin xu* syndromes include internal heat, they are also known as *xu* heat syndromes.

Yang xu syndromes are manifested by chills, cold extremities, tastelessness in the mouth, absence of thirst, pale complexion, spontaneous sweating, profuse and clear urine, loose stool, and pale tongue proper. Thus while *yang xu* syndromes indicate inadequate *yang qi*, they are also termed syndromes of *xu* cold.

Generally, symptoms characterized by excitation, restlessness, hyperactivity, and optimism belong to *yang* syndromes, while those characterized by inhibition, quietude, decline, and gloominess are *yin*.

Yang collapse and yin collapse syndromes: *Yang* and *yin* collapse syndromes are dangerous signs during the progress of a disease. *Yin* collapse indicates an excessive loss of vital essence and nutrient fluid. *Yang* collapse causes pathological changes and symptoms due to the profuse consumption of body *yang qi*. Both may occur at the final stage of some chronic diseases or may appear in the crisis stage of some acute diseases. Because of the interdepending relationship of *yin* and *yang*, a collapse of one could lead to the collapse of the other. Therefore, the occurrence of these syndromes might be simultaneous with only the difference of early or late appearance.

Besides the symptoms of primary disease, collapses of *yang* and *yin* are both manifested by different degrees of perspiration. The perspiration in *yin* collapse is characterized by a type of sticky hot sweat, accompanied by hot skin, warm hands and feet, thirst with preference for drinks, malar flush, and a thready, rapid, forceless pulse. These are signs of *yin* fluid exhaustion. *Yang* collapse perspiration is notable for dripping sweat, thin cold sweats, accompanied by aversion to cold, lying with the body curled up, cold extremities, listlessness, pale complexion, and feeble pulse, all of which are signs of *yang qi* prostration.

The syndromes of each of the eight principles are varied, but are closely related to each other in clinical application. For example, when differentiating syndromes of exterior and interior, the syndromes of cold, heat, *xu*, and *shi* are also involved; the differentiation of *xu* and *shi* syndromes is also involved with syndromes of cold, heat, exterior, and interior.

During the process of disease development, sometimes there will be non-conformity between the nature and the manifestation of a disease; for example, in syndromes of pseudo-cold and real heat, syndromes of real cold and pseudo-heat, etc. So attention should be paid to the pseudo-phenomena when a disease has developed to a serious stage. Differentiation of syndromes according to the eight principles should be used actively to prevent deception by the pseudo-phenomena of a disease.

Section 2
Differentiating Syndromes According to the *Zang-Fu* Organs

This is an important component of the differentiation of syndromes in traditional Chinese medicine. Differentiating diseases according to the theory of *zang-fu* organs involves analyzing and identifying the disease condition by collecting clinical data from the four diagnostic methods. Other methods of differentiating syndromes also finally use the theory of *zang-fu* organs, and clinically this method is closely related to other methods of differentiation according to the eight principles, etiology of *qi* and blood, etc. Following is a brief description of the main syndromes of each of the *zang-fu* organs:

1. Differentiating Syndromes of the Heart

Syndromes of heart qi xu and Heart yang xu: Palpitation and shortness of breath aggravated by exertion, spontaneous sweating, thready and weak pulse, and regular pulse or irregular intermittent pulse, are the basic symptoms of heart *qi* deficiency (*xu*) and heat *yang* deficiency (*xu*). If the above symptoms are accompanied with a pale and lusterless complexion, lassitude and a pale tongue proper with whitish coating, they are in the category of heart *qi* deficiency. If they are complicated with chills, cold extremities, fullness of the chest, pallor, and a pale or dark purplish tongue proper, they are considered as syndromes of the heart *yang* deficiency.

If heart *qi* or heart *yang* is insufficient, then the blood circulation is not promoted and shortness of breath aggravated by exertion will manifest. If heart *yang* is inadequate to restrict heart fluid, there will be spontaneous sweating. *Qi* deficiency leads to blood deficiency and weakness of *yang qi*, so disorders of blood circulation will manifest by thready, weak, irregular or regular intermittent pulses. Heart *qi* deficiency, or the failure of *yang qi* and blood to nourish the tongue, face and body, causes a pale and lusterless complexion, pale tongue proper, and lassitude. heart *yang* deficiency fails to warm the limbs, which causes chills and cold extremities. Failure of *yang qi* in the chest causes the improper circulation of *qi* and blood, manifesting a fullness in the chest and a dark purplish tongue proper.

Syndromes of heart blood deficiency and heart yin deficiency: Palpitation, insomnia, dream disturbed sleep and poor memory. If these symptoms are accompanied with a lusterless complexion, dizziness, pale tongue and lips, and a thready pulse, then these are heart blood deficiency syndromes. If the symptoms are complicated with irritability, thirst, feverish sensation of the palms and soles, tidal fever, night sweating, dry red tongue proper, and a thready rapid pulse, then these are heart *yin* deficiency syndromes.

The heart dominates the blood and its vessels, so heart blood deficiency and heart *yin* deficiency both cause malnourishment of the head region, manifesting as malnourishment of the mind, producing symptoms of palpitation, poor memory, insomnia, and dreamed disturbed sleep; malnourishment of the facial region, producing symptoms of lusterless complexion, pale tongue and lips; malnourishment of the brain, manifesting as dizziness and a thready weak pulse. Heart *yin* insufficiency also leads to heart *yang* preponderance and internal *xu* fire disturbances which cause irritability, feverish sensation of the palms, dry red tongue proper with scanty fluid, and thready rapid pulse.

Syndromes of heart fire preponderance: Ulcers of the tongue and mouth, anxiety, insomnia, thirst, yellowish urine, a red tongue tip, and rapid pulse.

The heart opens to the tongue. If there is a preponderance of heart fire, it flares up to attack the tongue causing ulceration. If heart fire causes internal disturbances, it first affects the mind, causing irritability and insomnia. A preponderance of heart fire consumes the body fluids, causing thirst, red tongue tip, and rapid pulse.

Stagnation of heart blood syndromes: Palpitation, paroxysmal pricking pain, or stuffy pain of the precardiac region referring to the shoulder and arm of the left side, cyanosis of the lips and nails, cold extremities, spontaneous sweating, dark red tongue proper, or purplish tongue proper with petechiae, thready rugged pulse, or regular and irregular intermittent pulse.

Obstruction of heart *yang* leads to unsmooth circulation of *qi* and blood, and the stagnation of blood in the vessels, causing palpitation and cardiac pain. The small intestine channel of the hand Taiyang is exterior and interior related to the heart channel, so the *qi* of the two channels affect each other, that is why cardiac pain is related to the shoulder and arm. The stagnation of heart blood may also bring on cyanosis of the lips and nails, dark red tongue proper, or purplish tongue proper with petechiae, thready rugged pulse, or regular and irregular intermittent pulse. Heart blood stagnation blocks the *yang qi* from spreading over the body surface and the four extremities, so cold extremities and spontaneous sweating result.

Phlegm fire heart-disturbing syndrome: Mental disorder, weeping and laughing without apparent reason (emotional liability), mania, redness of face, thirst, coarse breath, yellowish urine, yellow and sticky tongue coating, slippery, rapid, and forceful pulse.

Phlegm-fire disturbs the heart mind and exhausts the body fluid, so the above symptoms and pulses appear.

2. Differentiating Syndromes of the Liver

Syndromes of liver blood insufficiency: Dizziness and vertigo, distending pain, redness of the eyes and face, anxiety and hot temper, dryness of the eyes, blurred vision, night blindness, numbness of the limbs, spasm of the tendons and muscles, scanty menstrual flow or amenorrhea, pale tongue proper, and thready pulse.

Insufficiency of liver blood brings about malnutrition of the head and eyes, and manifests as dizziness, dryness of the eyes, and blurred vision. Consumption of liver blood causes malnourishment of the tendons, manifested by numbness of the limbs, and spasms of the tendons and muscles. The *chong* channel's "sea of blood" dries up due to an insufficiency of liver blood, so scanty menstrual flow or amenorrhea appears. Blood insufficiency also causes a pale tongue proper and a thready pulse.

Liver fire flare up syndromes: Dizziness, distending pain redness of the eyes and flushed face, irritability and irascibility, dryness and bitter taste in the mouth, deafness, ringing in the ears, burning pain of the costal and hypochondriac regions, yellowish urine, constipation or vomiting blood (hematemesis), and nose bleeds (epistaxis), red tongue proper with yellow coating, wiry and rapid pulse.

Liver fire flares up to attack the head and eyes causing dizziness, distending pain, redness of the eyes and flushed face, bitter taste and dryness in the mouth, deafness and ringing in the ears. Fire injures the liver causing a dysfunction of the *qi* flow and since the liver is related to emotional activities, depression and anger can result. As the liver channel passes through the costal and hypochondriac regions, it causes pain in these areas.

Liver fire exhausts the blood and injures the vessels, so hematemesis and epistaxis occur. Yellowish urine, constipation, yellow tongue coating, and a rapid pulse are also signs of excessive liver fire.

Liver qi stagnation syndromes: Fullness of the chest, mental depression, sighing, distending pain of the chest and hypochondrium, irascibility, anorexia, belching, abnormal bowel movements, irregular menstruation, dysmenorrhea, premenstrual distending pain of the breasts, thin and white tongue coating, and wiry pulse.

Stagnation of liver *qi* leads to the dysfunction of the liver causing an unrestrained flow of *qi*, so symptoms such as mental depression, fullness of the chest, irascibility, and sighing appear. Liver *qi* can also flow transversely to attack the stomach and spleen, causing disorders of the ascending and descending stomach and spleen *qi*. Symptoms of belching, anorexia, and abnormal bowel movements result. The liver stores blood, so liver *qi* stagnation will certainly affect menstruation causing irregularity, dysmenorrhea, or pre-menstrual distending pain of the breasts. A wiry pulse is also caused by liver *qi* stagnation.

Liver wind stirring syndromes: There are three conditions commonly seen in the clinic. a) Extreme heat stirring up endogenous wind, manifesting as high fever, convulsion, neck rigidity, contracture of the four limbs, opisthotonos, red tongue proper and a wiry rapid pulse. b) *Yin* deficiency leading to *yang* preponderance, this extreme *yang* then turns into wind and manifests as sudden temporary loss of consciousness (syncope), convulsion, deviated mouth and eyes, tongue rigidity, hemiplegia, wiry, slippery, and forceful pulse. c) Insufficiency of liver blood causes the malnutrition of tendons and muscles, and produces wind, manifesting as numbness of the limbs, tremor of muscles or spasms of the extremities, tremor of the hands, pale tongue proper, a wiry and thready pulse, etc.

The first condition is a group of *shi* syndromes caused by extreme heat producing wind, the wind and fire then stir each other. The second condition originates from a loss of liver and kidney *yin* which leads to liver *yang* preponderance and an upward flow of *qi* and blood. The root of this disease is therefore *xu*, but symptomatically the syndromes appear as *shi* type. The third condition is also a *xu* condition due to insufficiency of blood which leads to malnutrition of the tendons and muscles.

Stagnation of cold in the liver channel syndromes: Distending pain of the lower abdomen, swelling and distension of the testis with a bearing down pain, pain and contracture of the scrotum referring to the lower abdomen, a white slippery tongue, and a wiry slow pulse.

The liver channel curves around the external genitalia and

passes through the lower abdominal region. Pathogenic cold is characterized by contraction and stagnation when it inhabits the liver channel. This results in the stagnation of *qi* and blood and causes the above symptoms.

3. Differentiating Syndromes of the Spleen

Spleen failure to carry out transportation and transformation syndromes: Anorexia, abdominal distension after meals, lassitude, sallow complexion, feeble breathing, loose stool, pale tongue proper with white thin coating, retarded and weak pulse.

Spleen *xu* causes a failure of transportation and transformation, and insufficiency of *qi* and blood, so the above symptoms appear.

Sinking of spleen qi syndromes: Prolapse of the uterus, gastroptosis, nephroptosis, chronic diarrhea, feeble breathing, yellowish complexion, pale tongue proper with white coating, and *xu* type pulse.

Spleen *qi* should ascend, however, spleen *xu* causes the *qi* to sink. If the spleen *qi* is too weak to elevate the *zang-fu* organs, then the prolapse of internal organs and symptoms showing spleen *qi* insufficiency occur.

Spleen blood control failure syndromes: Excessive menstruation, uterine bleeding, hemotochezia, bloody urine, purpura, pale complexion, lassitude, pale tongue proper, and a thready weak pulse.

The spleen controls blood. If it is unable to carry out this function, then the extravasation of blood occurs, plus the bleeding symptoms mentioned above. Bleeding affects the function of transportation of *qi* and blood, resulting in a pale complexion, lassitude, a pale tongue proper, and a thready weak pulse, which are signs of *qi* and blood *xu* (deficiency).

Pathogenic damp invasion of the spleen syndromes: Distension and fullness of the epigastrium and abdomen, anorexia, stickiness in the mouth, heaviness of the head, absence of thirst, swelling of the face, eyes, and four extremities, loose stool, dysuria, excessive and thin leukorrhea, white and sticky tongue coating, and soft thready pulse.

The spleen is adverse to dampness, therefore excessive dampness is liable to affect spleen *yang* leading to a dysfunction of transportation and transformation, resulting in the symptoms of distension and fullness of the epigastrium and abdomen, and anorexia. Pathogenic damp, which is sticky and stagnant in nature, easily blocks the flow of *yang qi*, causing a sensation of heaviness of the head. If dampness and fluid pour into the skin and muscles, swelling of the face, eyes, and extremities occurs. If the spleen fails to remove the damp, the stool becomes loose and the urine abnormal. A white and sticky tongue coating and a soft thready pulse are signs of excessive pathogenic damp.

Spleen yang xu syndromes: Dull pain of the epigastrium and abdomen ameliorated by warmth, chills with cold extremities, poor appetite, loose stool, pale tongue proper with white coating, and deep, slow pulse.

Spleen *yang* deficiency causes the stagnation of cold in the middle *jiao*, obstructing the functions of *qi*. Warmth can remove the obstruction, so the pain of the epigastrium and abdomen is ameliorated. Deficiency of spleen *yang* leads to a dysfunction of transportation and transformation, thus the failure of spleen *yang* to warm the body surface and extremities, and the occurrence of anorenxia, and loose stool. A pale tongue proper with a white coating and a deep slow pulse are signs of *xu* cold.

Spleen and stomach damp heat syndromes: Yellow-orange complexion, distension and fullness of the epigastrium and abdomen, nausea, vomiting, poor appetite, aversion to greasy food, heaviness of the body, yellowish urine, loose stool profuse and yellowish leukorrhea, yellowish and sticky tongue coating, soft and rapid pulse.

Damp heat accumulates in the skin causing a yellow-orange complexion. It also blocks the middle *jiao* causing symptoms of distension and fullness of the epigastrium and abdomen, nausea, vomiting, anorexia, and version to greasy food. Excessive damp causes heaviness and tiredness of the body. Damp heat descending leads to profuse yellowish leukorrhea. Deep yellow urine, loose stool, yellowish and sticky tongue coating, and soft pulse are signs of excessive damp heat.

4. Differentiating Lun Syndromes

Qi Deficient of the Lung: Feeble coughing, shortness of breath, clear and thin sputum, feeble breathing, speaking in a low voice, spontaneous sweating, pale and lusterless complexion, lassitude, pale tongue proper with thin white coating, *xu* and forceless pulse.

The lung dominates *qi* and controls respiration, so *qi* deficiency causes a weak cough, shortness of breath, and feeble breathing. *Qi* deficiency of the lung also leads to a failure of lung *qi* descent causing an accumulation of body fluid with resulting phlegm. There are also symptoms of cough with thin sputum, spontaneous sweating, pale and lusterless complexion, lassitude, pale tongue proper with white and thin tongue coating, and *xu* type pulse.

Yin deficiency of the lung: Dry cough without sputum or with a little sticky sputum, dryness of the mouth and throat, hoarseness of voice, emaciation, dry red tongue proper, thready and forceless pulse. If *yin* deficiency leads to a preponderance of fire, there may be cough with bloody sputum, tidal fever, night sweating, malar flush, red tongue proper, and a thready rapid pulse.

The symptoms of lung *yin* deficiency are actually the manifestations of an insufficiency of lung *yin* fluid, i.e., dry cough without sputum, or cough with a little sticky sputum, dryness of the mouth and throat, hoarseness of voice, emaciation, dry red tongue proper, thready and forceless pulse. If *yin xu* fails to restrict *yang*, then *xu* fire is formed and flares up to damage the vessels of the lung, producing the symptoms of tidal fever, night sweating, malar flush, hematemesis, red tongue proper, thready rapid pulse.

Lung wind-cold retention syndromes: Cough, asthma, thin white sputum, absence of thirst, nasal obstruction, runny nose, chills and fever, no sweating, pain of the head and body, thin white tongue coating, superficial and tense pulse.

Exogenous pathogenic wind-cold obstructing the lung leads to the dysfunction of lung *qi* spreading and descending, causing symptoms of cough with thin white sputum. The lung opens into the nose, which is then also troubled by nasal obstruction or discharge. The lung dominates the skin and hair, when exogenous pathogenic wind and cold invade the lung leading to the dysfunction of defensive (*wei*) *qi*, the symptoms are an aversion to cold, fever, pain of the head and body, absence of sweat, thin white tongue coating.

Lung wind-heat invasion syndromes: Cough with yellowish and thick sputum, thirst, sore throat headache, fever, aversion to wind, yellowish and thin tongue coating, floating and rapid pulse.

The lung is attacked by exogenous pathogenic wind-heat, so the spreading and descending functions are affected, causing cough with a yellowish and thick sputum. Pathogenic heat consumes the body fluid, causing thirst. Wind and heat flow upward to cause a sore throat. Headache, fever, aversion to wind, yellowish and thin tongue coating, floating and rapid pulse are signs indicating wind-heat invasion of the defensive (*wei*) *qi* of the body surface.

Lung phlegm damp obstruction syndromes: Cough with excessive and white sticky sputum, expectoration, stuffiness of the chest, asthma, white sticky tongue coating, slippery pulse.

Pathogenic phlegm damp obstructing the lung leads to the impairment of *qi* circulation causing the above symptoms. White sticky tongue coating and slippery pulse are signs of pathogenic phlegm damp.

A long-standing obstruction of phlegm damp in the lung will

change into heat, blocking *qi* circulation and manifesting as asthmatic cough, stuffiness of the chest, etc. In addition, other symptoms may occur, such as cough with yellowish, sticky and thick sputum, or cough with bloody and pussy sputum. Fever, thirst, yellowish urine, constipation, red tongue proper with yellow sticky coating, and slippery pulse, are signs of heat syndromes.

5. Differentiating Syndromes of the Kidney

Kindey yang deficiency syndromes: Chilliness, cold extremities, aching and weakness of the lumbar region and knee joints, impotence, praecox ejaculation, excessive and thin leukorrhea, infertility, profuse and clear urine or enuresis, pale tongue proper with white coating, deep, slow and forceless pulse.

The kidney stores essence which is the original source of reproduction, therefore kidney *yang* deficiency will influence the genital system and sexual activities. Symptoms seen in men are impotence and praecox ejaculation, and in women excessive and clear leukorrhea, and infertility. The kidney dominates the bones and is the site of primary *yang qi* convergence. Insufficient *yang qi* of the kidney fails to warm and nourish the body and extremities, causing chilliness, aching and weakness of the lumbar region and knee joints. The kidney dominates water metabolism, so kidney *yang* deficiency causes a dysfunction of urinary bladder restriction, manifesting enuresis or profuse and clear urine. A pale tongue proper with white coating and a deep, slow and forceless pulse are signs of *yang* deficiency.

Kidney yin deficiency syndromes: Dizziness, vertigo, ringing in the ears, deafness, hair loss, loosening teeth, soreness and weakness of the lumbar region and knee joints, insomnia, poor memory, dryness of the throat, night sweating, feverish sensation of palms and soles, low fever, malar flush, red tongue proper, thready, rapid pulse, etc.

Yin deficiency produces internal heat, so symptoms such as low fever, malar flush, feverish sensation of the palms and soles, and night sweating occur. *Yin* deficiency also leads to insufficiency of body fluid manifested by dryness of the throat. Consumption of kidney *yin* causes soreness and weakness of the lumbar region and knee joints, hair loss and loosening teeth. *Yin* deficiency also causes the kidney to fail in its function of producing marrow, and with it filling out the brain. Manifestations are dizziness, vertigo, poor memory and insomnia. *Yin* deficiency is unable to nourish the upper orifices, and is manifested by ringing in the ears and deafness. Red tongue proper, and thready and rapid pulse are also signs of *yin* deficiency.

Kidney qi deficiency syndromes: Shortness and weakness of breath, asthmatic breathing aggravated by exertion, perspiration, cold extremities, swelling of the face, pale tongue proper, *xu* type pulse, etc.

The kidney dominates the reception of *qi*, so its weakness causes the *qi* to lose its function of controlling reception. The symptoms of shortness and weakness of breathing result. Asthmatic breathing aggravated by exertion is due to the consumption of *qi*. The *xu* condition of the kidney brings on *yang* deficiency leading to the weakness of *wei* (defensive) *qi*, so symptoms of perspiration appear. Cold extremities are due to *yang qi* failing to reach and warm the four extremities. *Yang* deficiency also has difficulty in promoting *qi* circulation and water metabolism, so there is swelling of the face. pale tongue proper and *xu* pulse are also signs of kidney *qi* deficiency.

Kidney xu leading to excessive water: General edema with greater severity in the lower extremities, abdominal distention, scanty urine, short breathing, cough and asthma with sputum gurgling in the throat, palpitations, asthma aggravated by exertion, chilliness and cold extremities, flabby tongue body with white coating and deep thready pulse.

The declining of kidney *yang* causes a dysfunction of the urinary bladder *qi* activity, manifesting as scanty urination. General edema is due to the water and fluid overflowing into the skin and muscles. Retention of water and fluid in the abdominal cavity gives rise to local distension. Excess water and fluid converts into phlegm, manifesting as cough and asthma with sputum gurgling in the throat. If water and fluid overflow upward they attack the heart and lung causing symptoms of palpitation and shortness of breath. *Yang* deficiency fails to warm and nourish the extremities, so it causes chilliness and cold extremities. Flabby tongue body, white tongue coating, deep and thready pulse are signs of *yang* deficiency causing an overflow of water and fluid.

Unconsolidated kidney qi syndromes: Frequent and clear urination, incontinence, dribbling of urine, nocturnal enuresis, involuntary seminal discharge without dreams, praecox ejaculatio, soreness and weakness of the lumbar region, wan complexion, pale tongue proper with white coating, thready and weak pulse.

The kidney stores essence, if kidney *xu* fails to consolidate the source of semen involuntary seminal discharge and praecox ejaculatio occur. Kidney *xu* causes the dysfunction of urinary bladder restriction seen in the symptoms of frequent and clear urination, dribbling of urine, incontinence, and nocturnal enuresis. The waist is the house of the kidneys, deficiency causes soreness and weakness of the lumbar region. Wan complexion, pale tongue proper with white coating, and thready weak pulse are signs of *yang xu* in the kidney.

Syndromes a, c, d, and e are based on the insufficiency of kidney *yang*. However, each has its own emphasis on pathological changes and clinical manifestations. The non-consolidation of kidney *qi* mainly indicates syndromes of *yang xu* of the kidney which causes uncontrollable seminal emissions and the dysfunction of the urinary bladder restriction. Kidney *yang xu* also leads to an inability to receive *qi* from the lung. Kindey *xu*, resulting in the overflow and subsequent retention of water, derives from dysfunction syndromes of the kidney, which normally controls water metabolism and *qi* activity. The declining of kidney *yang* also shows the hyndromes of hyperactive sexual function.

6. Differentiating Syndromes of the Small Intestine

Syndromes of shi heat in the small intestines: Scanty yellowish urine; burning pain of the urethra, or hematuria; ulceration and pain of the mouth and tongue; a feverish sensation with irritability in the chest.

The heart has an exterior and interior relationship to the small intestine, so a preponderance of heart fire will transmit to the small intestine resulting in *shi* heat syndromes of the small intestine.

7. Differentiating Syndromes of the Large Intestine

Large intestine damp-heat syndromes: Abdominal pain, dysentery or stool containing blood and pus, tenesmus, burning sensations of the anus, scanty and yellowish urine, yellow and sticky tongue coating, wiry, slippery and rapid pulse.

The retention of damp-heat in the large intestine causes a dysfunction of *qi* activity with resulting abdominal pain and tenesmus. Damp-heat injures the *qi* and blood of the intestinal tract, so dysentery, or bloody and purulent stool occur. Burning sensation of the anus is a characteristic manifestation of "downward pouring of damp-heat into the large intestine." Scanty yellowish urine, yellow sticky tongue coating, and wiry, slippery, and rapid pulse are signs of internal retention of damp-heat.

Large intestine fluid exhaustion: Constipation, difficult defecation of dry stools, dryness of the mouth and throat, red tongue proper with yellow and dry coating, rough or thready pulse.

Fluid exhaustion causes the large intestine to lose its moisture with resulting constipation. Dryness of the mouth and throat, red tongue proper with a yellow dry coating and a thready or rough pulse are all signs of fluid consumption.

8. Differentiating Syndromes of the Urinary Bladder

Syndromes damp of-heat in the urinary bladder. Frequency, urgency and pain of urination; dribbling urination; turbid urine of bloody and purulent urine; urine with stones; a yellow sticky tongue coating; and rapid pulse.

The accumulation of damp-heat in the urinary bladder blocks *qi* activity, causing dribbling urination. A downward driving of damp-heat into the urinary bladder brings about frequent, urgent and painful urination. Bloody or purulent urine is due to the injury of blood vessels by damp-heat.

9. Differentiating Syndromes of the Stomach

Loss and deficiency of stomach yin. Dryness of the mouth and throat, stomach-ache and hunger without desire to eat, dry stool, red tongue proper with scanty fluid, thready and rapid pulse.

Insufficiency of stomach *yin* makes the body fluid fail to support the upper organs, causing dryness of the mouth and throat. Insufficiency of stomach fluid leads to the dysfunction of stomach reception manifested by hunger without desire to eat. Deficiency of stomach *yin* also gives rise to the disturbances of *xu* fire, manifesting as stomach pain. Insufficiency of stomach *yin* causes dry stool. Red tongue proper with scanty fluid and a thready rapid pulse are signs of *yin* deficiency producing heat.

Preponderance of stomach fire. Burning pain of the epigastric region, vomiting, nausea, acid regurgitation, constipation, thirst with preference for cold drinks, swelling, pain, ulceration and bleeding of the gums, hunger with excessive eating, foul breath, red tongue proper with yellow coating, slippery and rapid pulse.

Accumulation of heat in the stomach leads to a dysfunction of *qi* activities resulting in a burning pain of the epigastrium. Preponderance of heat in the stomach consumes the *yin* of the stomach causing thirst with a preference for cold drinks. Since pathogenic fire accelerates food, there is hunger with excessive eating. Branches of the stomach channel travel up to the gum, therefore when pathogenic stomach heat flows upward, it causes welling, pain, ulceration and bleeding of the gums. An accumulation of stomach heat leading to a dysfunction of stomach *qi* descent causes foul breath, vomiting, nausea, and acid regurgitation. A red tongue proper with yellow coating and a slippery rapid pulse are signs of stomach heat.

Retention of Food in the Stomach:

Distension or pain in the epigastrium, foul belching, acid regurgitation, no desire to eat, vomiting, abnormal bowel movements, diarrhea or constipation, thick sticky tongue coating, and slippery pulse.

Retention of blood in the stomach blocks the *qi* activities of the middle *jiao*, so there is distension or pain in the epigastrium. Foul belching, acid regurgitation, no desire to eat, and vomiting are caused by a dysfunction of stomach *qi* descent, which then causes the upward flow of turbid *qi*. Retention of food in the stomach affects the transportation and transformation functions of the spleen, producing abnormal bowel movements, i.e., diarrhea or constipation. A thick sticky tongue coating and a slippery pulse are signs of food retention.

10. Differentiating Gall Bladder Syndromes

Phlegm disturbing the gall bladder. Dizziness, vertigo, bitter taste in the mouth, nausea, vomiting, irritability, insomnia, fright, fullness of the chest, sighing, slippery and sticky tongue coating, wiry pulse.

The gall bladder channel travels up to the head and eyes, so dizziness and vertigo are caused by pathogenic phlegm disturbing the brain along the course of the gall bladder channel. Internal phlegm disturbances lead to a restlessness of gall bladder *qi* resulting in irritability, insomnia, and fright. Stagnation of gall bladder *qi* affects the free flow of *qi*, this causes fullness of the chest and sighing. Since bile streams upward, there is a bitter taste in the mouth. *Qi* stagnation of the gall bladder also disturbs the stomach *qi*'s descent leading to nausea and vomiting. A sticky and slippery tongue coating and wiry pulse are signs of phlegm obstruction.

Section 3
Differentiating Syndromes According to the Theories of the Six Channels, Four Stages of *Wei*, *Qi*, *Ying* and *Xue*, and *Sanjiao*

The theories of the six channels, four stages of *wei*, *qi*, *ying* and *xue* are methods of differentiating syndromes of febrile diseases caused by exogenous pathogenic factors.

Differentiating syndromes according to the theory of six channels first appeared in the *Shang han lun* (*The Treatise on Febrile Diseases Caused by Exogenous Pathogenic Factors*) by Zhang Zhongjing of the Eastern Han Dynasty (25-220). In this book various clinical manifestations of febrile disease caused by exogenous pathogenic factors such as Taiyang syndromes, Yangming syndromes, Shaoyang syndromes, Taiyin syndromes, Shaoyin syndromes, and Jueyin syndromes are used to explain the location and nature of pathological changes, the strength and weakness of anti-pathogenic and pathogenic *qi*, and the tendency of disease development, as a guide for clinical treatment.

Differentiating syndromes according to the theory of four stages of *wei*, *qi*, *ying*, and *xue* was first put forward by Ye Tianshi, a Qing Dynasty (1644-1911) physician, in his book *Wan gan wen re pain* (*On Febrile Diseases Caused by Pathogenic Mild*

Heat). He classified the clinical manifestations of febrile diseases caused by pathogenic mild heat into four stage, *wei* (outer defensive) stage, *qi* (inner defensive) stage, *ying* (nutrient) stage, and *xue* (blood) stage. These are the four body strata used to explain the location and severity of pathological changes, and which form the basis of clinical treatment. Differentiating syndromes according to the theory of *sanjiao* was advocated by Wu Jutong, another Qing Dynasty physician. He summarized clinical manifestations of epidemic febrile diseases as having three areas: the upper, middle, and lower portions of the body cavity. These are also used to guide clinical treatment.

These three methods are not contradictory, rather they supplement each other's deficiencies. They can be used jointly to differentiate febrile diseases caused by exogenous pathogenic factors.

1. Differentiating Syndromes According to Six Channels Theory

Taiyang Diseases

A Taiyang disease is a pathological syndrome caused by exogenous pathogenic factors invading the body surface; it is also known as an exterior syndrome. Taiyang disease can be classified into syndromes of the Taiyang channel and syndromes of the Taiyang *fu* organ (urinary bladder).

1) Syndromes of the Taiyang channel: Aversion to cold, fever, pain and rigidity of the neck, thin white tongue coating, floating pulse.

Exogenous pathogenic factors attack the body surface injuring the defensive *yang qi* causing an aversion to cold. Fever is due to the obstruction of *yang qi*. Since the *qi* of the Taiyang channel is also affected, this results in headache, and neck pain and rigidity. A floating pulse indicates that pathological changes are exterior.

These are common manifestations of Taiyang exterior syndromes. On this basis, if they are accompanied by sweating, aversion to wind, floating and superficial pulse, they are known as wind stroke syndromes of Taiyang or exterior *xu* syndromes caused when the defensive *qi* is invaded by exogenous pathogenic wind. This leads to a disharmony between defensive and nutrient *qi*. If aversion to cold is not accompanied by sweating and a floating tense pulse, this is understood as Taiyang febrile syndrome caused by cold or exterior *shi* syndromes. In this case, exogenous pathogenic cold has obstructed the body surface and blocked the *yang qi* flow.

In addition, since the lung dominates the skin and hair, if exogenous pathogenic factors attack the body surface, lung *qi* will lead to dysfunction causing nasal obstruction, cough, asthma, etc.

2) The fu syndromes of Taiyang: The Taiyang *fu* organ syndromes are mainly due to a progression of Taiyang channel syndromes which are not cured when they are on the exterior, and then are transmitted along the channel into the urinary bladder. Taiyang *fu* syndromes are classified into water retention and blood retention syndromes.

Water retention syndromes: Fever, perspiration, irritability, thirst with or without preference for drinks, vomiting after drinking, and dysuria.

These syndromes are due to exogenous pathogenic factors being transmitted from the exterior to the interior, giving rise to *qi* activity dysfunctions in the urinary bladder. This further affects the body fluid flow leading to fluid retention and its sequence of irritability, thirst with preference for drinks, vomiting after drinking, and dysuria.

Blood retention syndromes: Pain and lump in the lower lateral abdomen, mania, normal urination.

Pain and lump in the lower lateral abdomen resulting from pathological heat transmitted along the Taiyang channel and mixing with blood in the lower *jiao*. Mental mania is caused by an upward disturbance due to blood retention and pathogenic heat. Since the disease location is in the blood of the lower *jiao*, the urinary bladder is not affected, thus there is normal urination.

Yangming Diseases

Yangming diseases are usually caused by exogenous pathogenic wind and cold which convert to heat and transmit directly into the interior, attacking the Yangming. They may also be due to delayed treatment causing body fluid consumption, which dries the stomach and intestines, resulting in constipation. Yangming diseases exhibit the greatest conflict between pathogenic and anti-pathogenic factors. They are also divided into syndromes of the Yangming channel and Yangming *fu* organ.

1) Yangming channel syndromes: Fever, perspiration, thirst with preference for drinking, irritability, yellow dry tongue coating, forceful pulse.

Pathogenic heat retained in the Yangming channel causes hyperactivity of heat in the stomach, manifesting as fever. Pathogenic heat forces the body fluid to flow outward, thus sweating occurs. This perspiration consumes fluids, so there is thirst with a preference for drinking. Irritability is due to heat disturbing the heart-mind. A dry yellow tongue coating is a sign of excessive heat injuring the body fluid. A forceful pulse indicates excessive heat and preponderant *yang*.

2) Yangming fu organ syndromes: Fever, tidal fever at dusk, sweating, constipation, fullness and pain of the abdomen (worse with pressure), irritability, delirium or even coma, yellow and dry tongue coating, or yellow coating with thorns, deep, forceful *shi* pulse.

Constipation is due to dryness of the intestine. The dysfunction of *qi* circulation in the *fu* organ causes a fullness and distending pain in the abdomen which is worse with pressure. Steaming of interior heat is the cause of fever and sweating. The Yangming *qi*, peaking at dusk, causes tidal fever when it contends with pathogenic factors. Irritability and delirium or even coma are caused by heat disturbing the heart-mind. Deep and *shi* pulse, and yellow and dry tongue coating with thorns are signs of interior *shi* heat leading to the insufficiency of body fluid.

Shaoyang Diseases

Shaoyang diseases are usually due to unrelieved Taiyang exterior syndromes that have been transmitted into the interior. There may be cases which have Taiyang diseases at the onset, so pathological changes are neither on the Taiyang exterior nor in the Yangming interior, but stay in between. They are known as semi-exterior/interior syndromes.

Main clinical manifestations: Bitter taste in the mouth, dryness of the throat, vertigo, alternate chills and fever, fullness of the chest and epigastric regions, poor appetite, irritability, vomiting, white slippery tongue coating, wiry pulse.

Pathogenic factors invade the Shaoyang and contend with anti-pathogenic *qi* in the region between the surface and the interior, so there are alternating chills and fever. The foot Shaoyang channel is distributed along the lateral side of the chest and hypochondriac region. Fullness of the chest and epigastric regions results from the obstruction of *qi* circulation after pathogenic factors invade the Shaoyang channel. *Qi* stagnation of the gall bladder may also affect the stomach, so poor appetite, irritability and vomiting occur. Fire of the gall bladder flares up to cause a bitter taste, dry throat, and vertigo. Wiry pulse and white slippery tongue coating are due to pathogenic heat hindering the Shaoyang.

Taiyin Diseases

Taiyin diseases are mostly due to pathogenic cold directly attacking the middle *jiao* of a constitutionally weak patient, or due to delayed treatment of diseases of the three *yang* channels thus damaging the *yang* of the middle *jiao*.

Main clinical manifestations: Abdominal distension, vomiting, anorexia, diarrhea with pain preferring warmth and pressure, thirst, pale tongue proper with white coating, slow or delayed pulse.

The nature of Taiyin diseases is *xu* cold of the middle *jiao*, and interior retention of cold damp. The spleen is responsible for the elevation of clean *qi*, while the stomach is responsible for the descent of turbid *qi*. The spleen also dominates the function of transportation and transformation of food, and the stomach controls the function of receiving food. Thus when the middle *jiao* is weak and attacked by pathogenic cold, the functions of transportation, transformation, and food reception become abnormal causing interior retention of cold damp manifesting the above symptoms.

Shaoyin Diseases

Shaoyin diseases may be due to direct attack of the Shaoyin by exogenous pathogenic factors when the body has *yang* deficiency and cold; or due to the transmission of pathogenic factors from other channels into the Shaoyin; or due to treatment employing a strong diaphoretic action that injures the *yang*. After invasion of the Shaoyin by pathogenic factors causing *yin* symptoms, a change into cold may occur. If *yang* symptoms occur they may transform into heat. Therefore Shaoyin diseases can be divided into Shaoyin syndromes of cold transformation and Shaoyin syndromes of heat transformation.

1). Cold transformation Shaoyin syndromes: Aversion to cold, sleeping with the knees drawn up, listlessness, cold extremities, loose stool with undigested food, vomiting, absence of thirst, preference for hot drinks, profuse and clear urine, pale tongue with white coating, deep and feeble pulse.

Shaoyin syndromes of cold transformation are the manifestations of heart and kidney *yang* deficiencies and interior retention of *yin* cold. Insufficient *yang qi* fails to warm and nourish the extremities resulting in cold extremities and sleep with the knees drawn up. Listlessness is due to the inability of *yang qi* to nourish the mind. Kidney *yang* deficiency is unable to warm the middle *jiao* leading to a dysfunction of the ascending and descending functions of middle *jiao qi*, resulting in loose stool with undigested food and vomiting. *Yang* deficiency unsuccessfully controls water, so there is profuse and clear urine. Absence of thirst, preference for hot drinks, pale tongue proper with white coating, and deep feeble pulse are all signs of *yang* deficiency and *yin* preponderance.

2) *Heat transformation Shaoyin syndromes*: Irritability, insomnia, dryness of mouth and throat, red tongue tip or deep red tongue proper with scanty tongue coating, deep, thready, and rapid pulse.

The patient usually has a *yin* deficiency. After pathogenic factors invade the Shaoyin, they are liable to transform into heat affecting kidney *yin*. A lessening of kidney *yin* (body fluid) prevents its upward flow to the heart and leads to hyperactivity of the heart fire. Symptoms of irritability, insomnia, dryness of the mouth and throat, deep red tongue, deep, thready, and rapid pulse occur.

Jueyin Diseases

Jueyin diseases indicate the last stage of disease transformation of the six channels. This disease condition is complex with syndromes of extreme heat or extreme cold, or syndromes of alternate cold and heat.

1) *Extreme cold syndromes*: Cold extremities, absence of fever, aversion to cold, pale tongue, and an extremely thready, feeble pulse that can hardly be felt.

Syndromes of extreme cold result from *yang xu* (deficiency) and excessive *yin*. So syndromes of extreme cold are also know as "coldness due to extreme *yin*."

2) *Extreme heat syndromes*: Coldness of extremities, irritability, feverish sensation, thirst, yellowish urine, yellowish tongue coating and slippery pulse.

Irritability, feverish sensation, thirst, yellowish urine, yellowish tongue coating and slippery pulse are signs of interior accumulation of heat. This interior accumulation causes a failure of the *yang qi* to warm and nourish the body surface. The resulting cold extremities are considered "coldness due to extreme *yang*," or "coldness due to extreme heat."

3) Coldness due to ascariasis syndromes: Cold limbs, *xiao ke* (general term for diseases with symptoms of frequent drinking of water, urination and bowel movements), a feeling of *qi* striking upward, pain and feverish sensation of the heart, hunger without appetite, vomiting ascariasis after eating food and serious diarrhea.

This condition is caused by parasitosis accompanied with mixed heat and cold. The symptoms of *xiao ke*, a feeling of *qi* striking upward, and pain and feverish sensation of the heart are heat syndromes. Hunger without appetite, vomiting ascariasis after eating, and serious diarrhea are cold syndromes. The mixture of heat and cold and the disharmony of *yin* and *yang* causes coldness of the limbs. Ascariasis disturbs the upper part of the body, manifesting irritability, and vomiting ascarids after eating.

2. Differentiating Syndromes According to the Theory of *Wei*, *Qi*, *Ying*, and *Xue*

This is a method of analyzing and judging the development of febrile diseases caused by exogenous pathogenic factors. *Wei* (outer defensive), *qi* (inner defensive), *ying* (nutrient), and *xue* (blood) are not only generalizations of the four types of febrile disease syndromes, but also a reflection of the four grades of severity of febrile diseases during their development.

Wei (Outer Defensive) Stage Syndrome
Wei (outer defensive) stage syndromes are seen at the onset of epidemic febrile diseases, the pathological changes occurring in the lung, and on the skin and hair. Clinical manifestations are characterized by the common exterior syndromes of fever and aversion to wind and cold.

Differentiation of Syndromes

Main clinical manifestations: Fever, a slight aversion to wind and cold, very little or no sweating, cough, headache, sore throat, slight thirst, a red tongue tip with thin white or slight yellowish tongue coating, floating and rapid pulse.

An attack of mild pathogenic heat on the body surface blocks the circulation of *wei* (defensive) *qi*, thus leading to dysfunction of the opening and closing of the pores and weakness of the defensive function of the body surface. Symptoms of fever, slight aversion to wind and cold, little or no sweating, and headache result. The lung dominates the skin and hair. Since the *wei qi* is blocked on the body surface, then the lung *qi* loses its function of spreading and descending *qi*, thus cough·and sore throat result. Thirst is caused by pathogenic heat consuming the body fluid. Red tongue tip with white thin or yellowish tongue coating, floating and rapid pulse are all signs indicating pathogenic mild heat attacking the *wei qi* of the body.

These symptoms are mainly manifestations of the loss of *wei qi*'s defensive function and also indicate a failure of the spread and descent of *qi*. If pathogenic factors mainly affect the skin and hair, that is, the body surface, then they are characterized by fever, thirst, and sore throat. If the lung is mainly affected, the chief complaint will be cough and sore throat.

Qi (Inner Defensive) Stage Syndrome

Syndromes of the *qi* (inner defensive) stage are the syndromes of interior heat due to the inner defense being invaded by pathogenic heat. In this case the anti-pathogenic *qi* and the pathogenic factor are very strong, resulting in hyperactivity of *yang* heat. Clinical manifestations are fever and no fear of cold.

Since the affected location alters after pathogenic heat is transmitted into the interior, the syndromes of the *qi* stage can then be classified into different types as follows:

1) Mild heat in the lung: Fever, perspiration, thirst, cough, asthma, chest pain, red tongue proper with yellow coating, rapid pulse.

Preponderance of interior heat causes fever, rapid pulse, and red tongue proper with yellow coating. Interior heat steams the body fluid bringing on perspiration and thirst. Retention of pathogenic heat in the lung leads to the dysfunction of lung *qi*'s spread and descent, so cough, asthma, and chest pain occur.

2) Accumulation of pathogenic heat in the chest and diaphragm: Fever, irritability, depression, restlessness, red tongue proper, slight yellowish tongue coating, thirst, constipation, rapid pulse.

Retention of heat inside the body causes fever. Pathogenic heat disturbs the mind, so irritability and restlessness result. Pathogenic heat consumes the body fluid resulting in thirst and constipation. Red tongue proper with a slightly yellowish coating, and rapid pulse are signs of excessive pathogenic heat.

3) Heat transmitted into the stomach: High fever, thirst with preference for cold drinks, profuse sweating, anxiety, dry and yellowish tongue coating, full and forceful pulse.

The pathogenesis and differentiation of *qi* stage syndromes is the same as for the Yangming channel syndromes. The only difference is the slower development of the disease condition after the invasion of pathogenic cold is transmitted from the Taiyang into the Yangming, while the transmission of pathogenic mild heat into heat is faster after it enters into the interior.

4) Retention of pathogenic heat in the liver and gall bladder: Retching, bitter taste in the mouth with thirst, irritability, insomnia, hypochondriac pain, yellowish tongue coating, wiry and rapid pulse.

Disharmony of *qi* circulation in the liver and gall bladder channels is due to interior heat retention in the liver and gall bladder. This causes hypochondriac pain, bitter taste in the mouth and a wiry pulse. Stagnation of heat in the liver and gall bladder affects the stomach, causing retching. Pathogenic heat disturbing the heart and mind brings on irritability and insomnia. A yellowish tongue coating and thirst are signs of excessive pathogenic heat.

5) Retention of pathogenic mild heat in the intestine: There are two different groups of clinical manifestations as follows.

a) Dryness of the intestine causing constipation with manifestations being the same as syndromes of the Yangming *fu* organs.

b) Heat in the intestine leading to diarrhea, a burning sensation around the anus, thirst, yellowish and dry tongue coating, rapid pulse.

Descending heat in the intestine causes a dysfunction of transportation and transformation, thus diarrhea and a burning sensation around the anus result. Pathogenic heat consuming the body fluid produces thirst. Yellowish tongue coating and rapid pulse are signs of excessive pathogenic heat.

Ying (Nutrient) Stage Syndromes

The syndromes of the *ying* (nutrient) stage occur when pathogenic mild heat is transmitted into the superficial layer of the blood. *Ying* is a component of the blood, so the disease location is actually in the heart and pericardium. Pathological characteristics show the injury of nutrient *yin* and the disturbance of heart-mind.

1) Pathogenic heat injuring nutrient yin: Fever (worse at night), irritability, insomnia, or even coma and delirium, recessive rashes, slight thirst, deep red tongue proper, thready and rapid pulse.

Pathogenic mild heat invades deeply into the *ying* stage, thus scorching and injuring the nutrient *yin* and leading to insufficiency of blood, so the fever worsens at night and a rapid thready pulse results. Pathogenic heat steams nutrient *yin* causing a slight thirst. Heat disturbs the mind leading to irritability, insomnia, or even coma and delirium. Pathogenic heat causes a disorderly flow of blood, thus a recessive, deep red tongue proper manifests.

2) Heat attacking the pericardium: Fever, coma, delirium, deep red tongue proper, rapid pulse. After pathogenic heat attacks the pericardium, it disturbs the heart-mind bringing on fever, coma, and delirium. A deep red tongue proper is a sign of heat in the blood. Rapid pulse indicates excessive heat.

Xue Stage Syndromes

Syndromes of the *xue* (blood) stage denote pathogenic mild heat invading the blood to the deepest stage. The pathological changes are mainly in the liver and kidney. Clinical manifestations are characterized by heat in the blood causing disorderly flow, stirring up of wind and heat, and injury of body *yin*.

1) Heat in the blood causing disorderly flow: Hemorrhage (including hematemesis, epistaxis, bloody stools, purpura, and vaginal bleeding), blood of a dark red or dark purple color, fever (worse at night), irritability, insomnia, feverish sensation of the palms and soles, deep red tongue proper, and rapid pulse.

Extreme heat in the blood stage forces a disorderly flow of the blood causing hemorrhage. Blood of a dark red or dark purple color indicates heat. Fever, worse at night, and a feverish sensation of the palms and soles are both signs of heat in the blood causing *yin* deficiency. Irritability and insomnia result from heat disturbing the heart-mind. A deep red tongue proper and a rapid pulse are the manifestations of extreme heat in the blood.

2) Heat in the liver stirring up wind: Headache, dizziness, redness of the eyes, irritability, fever, thirst, stiffness of the neck and back, contracture of the four extremities, deep red tongue proper, wiry and rapid pulse.

Headache, redness of the eyes, dizziness are caused by heat in the liver channel. Irritability and thirst result from pathogenic mild heat consuming the body fluid. Extreme heat exhausts the *yin* fluid of the body, thus the blood fails to nourish the tendons with resulting stiffness of the neck and back, and contracture of the four limbs. A deep red tongue proper, and a wiry rapid pulse are signs of heat in the blood of the liver channel.

3) Heat in the blood injures yin: Fever, flushed face, heat of the palms and soles, dryness of the mouth, listlessness, deafness, *xu* and forceless pulse, accompanied by irritability, insomnia, protracted fever at dusk, chilliness in the early morning, no sweating after the fever subsides, red tongue proper with scanty coating, thready and rapid pulse.

Hot palms and soles, flushed face, dryness of the mouth, and deafness are all signs of *yin* deficiency and *yang* floating upward. Listlessness and *xu* pulse are caused by the insufficiency of essence and blood. Irritability and insomnia are due to *yin* deficiency producing a preponderance of fire which disturbs the heart-mind. No sweating after fever subsides, fever at dusk, and chilliness in the early morning are characteristics of *yin* deficiency producing heat.

4). *Perishing of yin and excessive loss of fluid*: Slim limbs, withered lips and shrunk tongue, dryness of gums, depressed eyes, unconsciousness, flushed cheeks, coldness of extremities, squirming fingers, feeble and unfelt pulse, or even convulsion.

Atrophy and dryness of the limbs, lips, and tongue, dryness of the gums, and depressed eyes are manifestations of perishing *yin* and excessive loss of fluid. Unconsciousness, feeble and unfelt pulse are signs showing complete exhaustion of *yin* fluid. Flushed cheeks, and cold extremities are signs of a heat nature showing the internal draining of *yin* fluid leading to the upward floating of *ying qi*, and a failure of *yang qi* to warm and nourish the four extremities. Squirming fingers indicate malnourishment of the tendons due to the internal draining of *yin* fluid, thus causing an internal stirring of *xu* wind.

3. Differentiating Syndromes According to the *Sanjiao* Theory

Differentiating syndromes according to the theory of *sanjiao* is a method of analyzing damp-heat syndromes in febrile diseases caused by exogenous pathogenic factors. Damp-heat syndromes are caused by exogenous pathogenic damp and heat, so the disease duration is long and the condition is complicated. Pathological changes are mainly in the middle *jiao*, especially concentrated in the spleen and stomach. At the early stage of damp-heat diseases there is no clear margin between *wei* (outer defensive) stage, and *qi* (inner defensive) stage. Also, before damp-heat is transformed into dryness, it may be transformed into *ying* (nutrient) stage, and *xue* (blood) stage. So it is difficult to differentiate damp-heat diseases by using the theory of *wei*, *qi*, *ying*, and *xue*. Generally, pathogenic damp and heat spread through all the upper, middle, and lower *jiao* to obstruct the circulation of *qi*, and block the smooth transportation and transformation of water and fluid. Thus, the method of differentiating syndromes according to the theory of *sanjiao* is used to analyze these diseases.

The syndromes of the upper, middle, and lower *jiao* are generalizations of the three kinds of symptom-complex, and a reflection of disease development from upper to lower, from superficial to deep, and from mildness to severity.

Damp-Heat in the Upper Jiao

Damp-heat in the upper *jiao* indicates the early stage of pathogenic injury. The main pathological changes are in the lung and body surface.

Main clinical manifestations: Severe aversion to cold, little or no fever, no sweating, heaviness and pain of the body, distending pain of the head, deafness, dull mind, indifferent emotions, hypersomnia, poor appetite, white sticky tongue coating, soft and weak pulse.

Damp is a *yin* pathogenic factor which attacks *yang qi* easily, so there is severe aversion to cold and a slight fever. Pathogenic damp obstructing the body surface muscles causes an absence of sweating and pain. Pathogenic damp is characterized by heaviness and turbidity, so the manifestations of heaviness of the body and distending pain of the head occur. Pathogenic damp misting of clear *yang* results in deafness, dull mind, indifferent emotions and hypersomnia. Poor appetite is caused by the retention of damp in the spleen and stomach. A white sticky tongue coating and a soft weak pulse are signs of excessive damp.

Damp-Heat in the Middle Jiao

Damp-heat in the middle *jiao* transmits from the upper *jiao*. The main pathological changes show the disturbance of damp on *qi* activities, and abnormal ascending and descending of middle *jiao qi*.

Main clinical manifestations: Fever, stuffiness and distension of the chest and epigastric region, anorexia, loose stools, scanty and yellowish urine, light yellow color of the face and eyes, grayish, pale and slightly yellow tongue coating, dull mind, coldness of the lower legs, and soft pulse.

Damp mixed with heat causes fever. Damp also obstructs the *qi* activities and disturbs its function of ascending and descending, so stuffiness and distension of the chest and epigastric region, anorexia, and loose stools occur. Steaming of damp and heat causes a light yellow face and eyes. *Yang qi* fails to spread over the four extremities due to a blockage of clear *yang* by damp, so a dull mind, and coldness of the lower legs result. Grayish, pale, and slightly yellow tongue coating, and a soft pulse are signs of excessive damp-heat.

Damp-Heat in the Lower Jiao

Damp-heat in the lower *jiao* arises from the middle *jiao*. The main pathological changes are characterized by problems of the urinary bladder and large intestine.

Retention of damp in the urinary bladder: Dysuria, distending pain and dizziness of the head, fullness and stuffiness of the epigastric and abdominal regions, grayish-white and yellow-sticky tongue coating, unsmooth bowel movements, and soft pulse.

Retention of dampness deranges the *qi* activities of the urinary bladder, manifesting as dysuria. Distending pain and dizziness of the head, and fullness and stuffiness of the epigastric and abdominal regions are caused by the failure of *yang qi* to ascend because of the spreading of damp-heat through the upper, middle, and lower *jiao*. Unsmooth bowel movements are the result of damp-heat retention in the large intestine. Grayish-white, yellow-sticky tongue coating, and a soft pulse are signs of excessive internal damp-heat.

Retention of damp in the large intestine: Constipated stool, fullness of the lower abdomen, distension of the head, stuffiness of the epigastrium, grayish and yellow-sticky tongue coating, and soft pulse.

Grayish and yellow-sticky tongue coating, and soft pulse indicate interior retention of excessive damp-heat. Distension of the head, and stuffiness of the epigastrium indicate damp-heat remaining in the upper, middle, and lower *jiao*, in which the *qi* activities of the *sanjiao* are blocked. Constipation and fullness of the lower abdomen are due to the stagnation of dampness disturbing the large intestine.

Chapter 8
Therapeutic Principles

Therapeutic principles are the basis for guiding clinical practice. They include *biao* (branch) and *ben* (root), that is, the principle of treating a disease by analyzing both its root cause and symptoms. Thus, factors such as climatic and seasonal conditions, geographic localities, and the patient's personal conditions must be considered in treatment, along with strengthening the *zheng qi* (the patient's body resistance or anti-pathogenic factors) and dispelling the *xie qi* (pathogenic factors).

1. The Principle of *Biao* and *Ben*

Biao and *ben* are contrasting concepts used to indicate the primary and secondary relationships of contradictory sides in various kinds of diseases and syndromes. For example, body resistance (or anti-pathogenic factors) are considered *ben* (root) while pathogenic factors are *biao* (branch); etiology is *ben*, symptom is *biao*; primary disease is *ben*, secondary disease is *biao*; pathological changes of internal organs are *ben*, body surface is *biao*, etc.

The principle of *biao* and *ben* is used in traditional Chinese medicine to treat the symptoms at the acute stage and to treat the root of disease at the chronic stage. If *biao* and *ben* have the same severity, treatment should then be applied to both *ben* (root cause) and *biao* (symptoms).

2. Strengthening the *Zheng Qi* and Dispelling *Xie Qi*

Zheng qi is the ability of body resistance against disease. *Xie qi* are the pathogenic factors. Strengthening the *zheng qi* and dispelling *xie qi* are two differing therapeutic principles. Generally, strengthening the *zheng qi* is used where body resistance is weak and pathogenic factors are not strong; dispelling *xie qi* is applied to cases which have excessive pathogenic factors, and also an unweakened body resistance. First, strengthening *zheng qi* and then dispelling *xie qi* is used in cases where the *zheng qi* and *xie qi* are not weakened. The simultaneous strengthening of *zheng qi* and dispelling of *xie qi* is applied in cases of weak body resistance where pathogenic factors are in excess. When this principle is employed, one must differentiate between what is primary and what is secondary. In strengthening *zheng qi*, allow for unforeseen pathogenic factors, and when dispelling pathogenic factors, do not influence the body resistance. It is necessary to make the principles of "strengthening body resistance" and "dispelling pathogenic factors" complement each other.

3. Principle of Treatment Based on Climatic and Seasonal Conditions, Geographic Localities, and Patient's Personal Conditions

Disease is the outcome of the struggle between body resistance and pathogenic factors. Therefore, in the treatment of a disease certain factors and conditions should be considered, that is, time (seasonal and climatic conditions), place (geographical location and environment), and personal characteristics (living customs, age, sex, and body constitution). In the clinical application of medicinal herbs these factors are also very important. This is an important therapeutic principle guiding clinical practice in traditional Chinese medicine. Examples follow:

In summer, the surface pores on the body are open or loose, while in winter they are closed and tight. If the body is affected by the same exogenous pathogenic wind and cold both in summer and winter then pungent drugs having a warming property of relieving exterior syndromes should not be administrated in summer, but should be used in large dosage in winter. Because summer is humid, the pathogenic factors which cause diseases in this season always mix with damp. Therefore, medicinal herbs used for summer diseases should be combined with herbs having properties of dissolving or removing damp.

The weather in mountainous regions and on plateaus is dry and cold, medicinal herbs having cold, cool, bitter, or dry properties should not be prescribed in large doses. While the climate in low-lying country is warm and humid, so drugs having cool and damp dissolving properties can also be used in large dosages.

Children have a body constitution of young and tender *yang*, for which *qi* and blood are not yet abundant, and a flourishing vitality. The vitality of aged people, however, is declining and *qi* and blood are insufficient. Therefore both children and elderly patients should not be prescribed drugs having strong properties, nor be given large dosages.

Obese patients are liable to have diseases caused by internal pathogenic damp, so drugs with cool, moist properties must not be given. Most thin patients are suffering from illness due to pathogenic fire, thus medicinal herbs with warm, dry properties are not suitable.

The same disease, but with different sexes, different physiological characteristics, and different body constitutions should be treated accordingly.

Chinese medical theory, as a product of traditional Chinese culture, reflects an extraordinary sensitivity toward Nature. Throughout the world, traditional Chinese medicine is praised for its holistic attitude in the understanding and curing of disease. With a 2,000-year written tradition, Chinese medical culture has accumulated an impressive body of theoretical and practical experience.

In this introductory volume we have presented the basic elements of Chinese medical theory in a systematic way designed for the English language reader. Our aim is to provide our reader with a "short cut" through the complexities of Chinese medical theory. The other volumes in this series will build upon the theoretical foundations set in this volume.

ENDNOTES

1. *Suwen*, Chapter 5.
2. *Suwn*, Chapter 6
3. *Suwn*, Chapter 5.
4. *Suwen*, Chapter 5.
5. *Suwen*, Chapter 25.
6. *Suwen*, Chapter 3.
7. *Suwen*, Chapter 5, *Yin-yang ying-xiang da-lun.*
8. *Leijing tuyi*, Chapter 1, *Wuxing tunglun.*
9. *Suwen*, Chapter 67, *Wuyunqi dalun.*
10. *Suwen*, Chapter 5.
11. See Table 1 for a list of the five colors, tastes, and tones.
12. *Nanjing*, Question 77.
13. *Suwen*, Chapter 11, *Wuzang bielun.*
14. *Suwen*, Chapter 44, *Wei lun.*
15. *Suwen*, Chapter 9.
16. *Lingshu*, Chapter 8.
17. *Lingshu*, Chapter 9.
18. *Suwen*, Chapter 74, *Zhizhenyao dalun.*
19. *Suwen*, Chapter 44.
20. *Suwen*, Chapter 17.
21. *Wang Bin's Annotations on the Suwen*, Chapter 10.
22. *Suwen*, Chapter 74.
23. *Wang Bin's Annotations on the Suwen*, Chapter 10.
24. *Suwen*, Chapter 10.
25. *Suwen*, Chapter 17.
26. *Suwen*, Chapter 4.
27. *Suwen*, Chapter 1.
28. *Suwen*, Chapter 1.
29. *Suwen*, Chapter 34.
30. *Suwen*, Chapter 10.
31. *Lingshu*, Chapter 18.
32. *Suwen*, Chapter 12.
33. *Lingshu*, Chapter 71.

Endnotes

34. *Lingshu*, Chapter 30.
35. *Suwen*, Chapter 26.
36. *Lingshu*, Chapter 47.
37. *Suwen*, Chapter 56.
38. *Cun* is a unit of Chinese measurement, one meter equals 30 *cun*. But when locating a point from physical landmarks, a system of unit measurement called *cun* is also used. The length of a *cun*, in this case, is relative to the physical proportions of the individual being measured.
39. *Suwen*, Chapter 44.
40. *Suwen*, Chapter 56.
41. *Suwen*, "On Febrile Disease" Section.
42. *Suwen*, "On Acupuncture Techniques."
43. *Suwen*, Chapter 29, says, "When wind invades the body, it attacks the upper region first."
44. *Suwen*, Chapter 42.
45. *Suwen*, Chapter 5.
46. *Suwen*, Chapter 29.
47. *Lingshu*, Chapter 28.

图书在版编目(CIP)数据

中医基础理论/耿俊英, 苏志红著
－北京: 新世界出版社, 1996.2 重印
ISBN 7－80005－114－5

Ⅰ.中…
Ⅱ.①耿…②苏
Ⅲ.中医医学－基础
Ⅳ.R22

中医基础理论

耿俊英　苏志红　著

＊

新世界出版社出版

(北京百万庄路 24 号)

北京大学印刷厂印刷

中国国际图书贸易总公司发行

(中国北京车公庄西路 35 号)

北京邮政信箱第 399 号　邮政编码 100044

1990(英文)第一版　1996 年第二次印刷

ISBN 7－80005－114－5

02400

14－E－2519P